Expert Guide to

ONCOLOGY

For a catalogue of publications available from ACP–ASIM, contact:

Customer Service Center
American College of Physicians–American Society of Internal Medicine
190 N. Independence Mall West
Philadelphia, PA 19106-1572
215-351-2600
800-523-1546, ext. 2600

Visit our Web site at www. acponline.org

EXPERT GUIDE TO
ONCOLOGY

JACOB D. BITRAN, MD

Director, Division of Hematology/Oncology
Lutheran General Hospital and Cancer Care Center
Park Ridge, Illinois

American College of Physicians
Philadelphia, Pennsylvania

Clinical Consultant: David R. Goldmann, MD, FACP
Acquisitions Editor: Mary K. Ruff
Manager, Book Publishing: David Myers
Administrator, Book Publishing: Diane McCabe
Production Supervisor: Allan S. Kleinberg
Production Editor: Victoria Hoenigke
Editorial Assistant: Alicia Dillihay
Interior Design: Patrick Whelan
Cover Design: Elizabeth Swartz

Printed in the United States of America
Composition by Fulcrum Data Services, Inc.
Printing/binding by Versa Press

American College of Physicians (ACP) became an imprint of the American College of Physicians–American Society of Internal Medicine in July 1998.

Library of Congress Cataloging-in-Publication Data

Bitran, Jacob D.
    Expert guide to oncology / Jacob D. Bitran.
        p.   ;   cm. – (Expert guide series)
    Includes bibliographical references.
    ISBN 0-943126-88-6
        1. Oncology. 2. Cancer. I. Title
    [DNLM: 1. Neoplasms. QZ 200 B624e 2000]
    RC254.B55 2000
    616.99'4

                                                              99-044526

The authors and publisher have exerted every effort to ensure that drug selection and dosage set forth in this manual are in accord with current recommendations and practice at the time of publication. In view of ongoing research, occasional changes in government regulations, and the constant flow of information relating to drug therapy and drug reactions, the reader is urged to check the package insert for each drug for any change in indications and dosage and for added warnings and precautions. This care is particularly important when the recommended agent is a new or infrequently used drug.

00 01 02 03 04/9 8 7 6 5 4 3 2 1

Preface

Cancer is the second leading cause of death for adults in the United States. As the U.S. population ages and as the number of deaths from cardiovascular disease continues to decline, sometime early in the new millennium cancer will overtake heart disease as the leading cause of death. Therefore medical students, physicians-in-training, and practicing physicians must obtain a better understanding of the biology, genetics, and diagnostic work-up of cancer, oncologic emergencies, and the palliative care of patients with cancer.

The purpose of this text is to impart, through the use of didactic material and case histories, the essentials of clinical oncology so that the aforementioned medical students, physicians-in-training, and practicing physicians may better care for patients with malignant diseases. The case histories, a key component of the ACP-ASIM Expert Guides series, use clinical situations commonly encountered by internists to discuss the diagnosis and treatment of typical patients.

Cancer therapies have changed over the past two decades and will continue to evolve. Although detailed information on the many types of cancer treatment is beyond the scope of this volume, important state-of-the-art therapies are described and analyzed. Here, in one concise volume, is the information internists need to know about cancer and its treatment.

Jacob D. Bitran, MD

Introduction

As we enter the new millennium, physicians in the United States will be faced with the dilemma of attempting to provide care to an aging population. Rates of cardiovascular disease, degenerative neurologic disorders, and malignancies will increase as our population ages. Elderly patients will no doubt be more computer savvy as a group than those at present and have access to a wider variety of on-line medical literature, receiving information via the Internet that is accurate at times and inaccurate at others. Even today, it is not unusual for patients to come to a doctor's office with a print-out of the latest information on a particular illness and to raise questions about relevant clinical trials and therapies.

Clearly, the future will challenge physicians. As always, there will be the responsibility of making an accurate diagnosis and providing the best possible medical care. But also, because of the additional information and misinformation that patients will bring to the office and consequently the treatments and therapies they will expect, physicians will need additional patience and tact. When discussing a patient's disease and treatment options, a physician will also have to be an educator, providing information, reinforcing truths, and dispelling myths about illnesses.

Unfortunately, cancer will likely still be a prevalent disease in the new century. Although we hope that someday cancer, like tuberculosis, will become a disease of a bygone era, the sad reality is that, for now, cancer is a disease that all physicians must be prepared to confront. All physicians must be knowledgeable about cancer because it is a disease that transcends specialties. Internists and primary care physicians in particular must be informed about cancer. It is the internist/primary care physician who in almost all cases makes the diagnosis, stages the cancer, and ensures that the appropriate referral is made at the appropriate time. It is also the internist/primary care physician who, together with the surgeon, surgical oncologist, radiation oncologist, and medical oncologist, continues the surveillance of the patient for recurrent disease. It is the internist/primary care physician who must be able to recognize and know how to treat the long-term complications of cancer therapy. It is the internist/primary care physician who is first approached and questioned by patients with cancer about treatment recommendations made by a specialist. The internist/primary care physician is also the person who most often helps patients sort through the maze of information and the overload of literature found in an Internet search of the disease. Finally, it is the internist/primary care physician who often directs end-of-life care.

The purpose of this book is to demystify cancer medicine and provide internists, who play such a significant role in the care of the patient with cancer, with a basic knowledge of clinical oncology. This knowledge will allow internists and primary care physicians to address the needs of their cancer patients and to provide the framework for dialogue with their colleagues who specialize in oncology and hematology.

Jacob D. Bitran, MD

Contents

Chapter 1

The Pathogenesis of
Malignant Transformation

Benign and malignant tumors (neoplasia) arise as a result of unregulated cellular growth and/or a failure of the programmed cell death pathway (apoptosis). Transformation of a normal cell into one that is malignant is a multi-step process in which exposure to a chemical or an environmental agent initiates chromosomal damage. The resultant malignant single cell over time develops into a neoplastic clone. This mutagenic process is called *initiation*. The survival of this transformed neoplastic single cell requires *promoters*, chemicals, proteins, or agents that alone have little to no carcinogenic potential. At this stage, growth may be reversible. Mechanisms that lead to regression include immunologic surveillance and/or activation of programmed cell death pathways. *Progression* implies the irreversible growth of this neoplastic clone. An example of this multi-step process is the initiation of colonic polyps and their progression to colonic cancer as shown in Figure 1-1. In this figure, unregulated growth of the colonic epithelium (polyps) results from mutational events in colonic cellular DNA, such as an interstitial deletion of the short arm of chromosome 5 (5p–). Further mutational events such as c-*myc* and K-*ras* activation causes further transformation into small and, subsequently, large polyps (adenomas). Increasing mutational events, such as a mutated p53 gene on the short arm of chromosome 17 or allelic loss on the long arm of chromosome 18 (deleted in colon cancer gene [*DCC*]), ultimately create an invasive colon cancer.

A malignant tumor may be thought of as having compartments of cells (Fig. 1-2). At any point in the growth of a tumor, differing proportions of

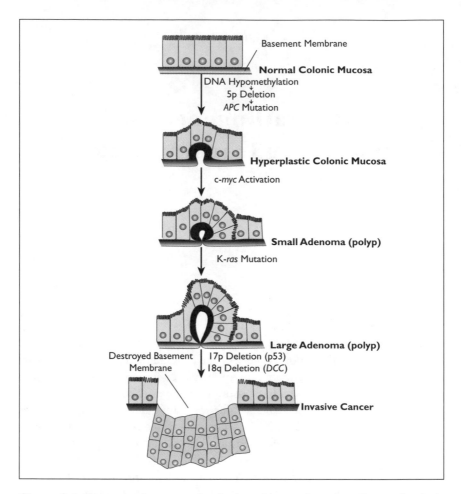

Figure 1-1 The molecular events that lead to the transformation of normal colonic mucosa to colonic polyps to invasive colon cancer.

cells may be in cell cycle, resting or moving from the resting compartment into cell cycle and vice versa. The nonproliferating compartment of cells accounts for tumor bulk. Small tumors have a greater percentage of cells in cell cycle than do large ones, which generally have few cells in cycle and therefore have a lower proliferative activity. Tumor growth occurs in a Gompertzian fashion, as shown in Figure 1-3. An initial exponential phase of growth is followed by a plateau phase, when cell death equals the rate of new daughter cell formation. Although the Gompertzian curve may be a reasonable model of tumor growth for leukemia and lymphomas, it may not accurately describe the growth and "dormancy" that characterizes many epithelial malignancies such as breast cancer and colonic cancer.

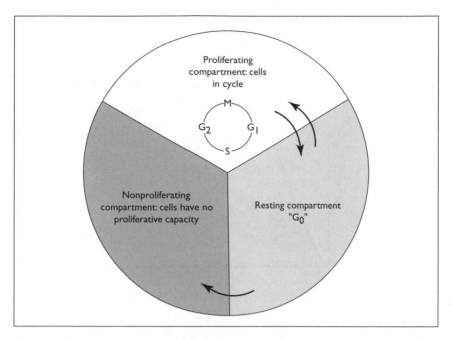

Figure 1-2 The cellular compartments within a malignant tumor mass. The proliferating compartment is the one in cell cycle.

The growth of these primary malignancies and metastatic foci may not be linear even when they are small. Growth may occur in spurts, followed by a latency period. A better model for explaining tumor growth may be the "chaos theory." In this model, some of the variables that govern growth (Table 1-1) include pro-apoptotic and anti-apoptotic factors, pro-angiogenesis and anti-angiogenesis factors, and the local "cytokine and steroid soup" in the extracellular matrix that an individual tumor is exposed to. All of these variables taken together create a dynamic equilibrium that governs local tumor growth. Inherent in chaos theory is that small alteration in these variables can have far-reaching effects on growth. Moreover, the theory may also explain dormancy or late relapses on the basis of a change in the dynamic equilibrium that favors growth as opposed to inhibiting it.

During the process of growth, a malignant tumor mass requires vasculature blood supply for the tumor to exceed 1 to 2 mm. Cancer cells have the ability to synthesize and secrete *angiogenic factors* that are vital in establishing capillary networks. In parallel to the process of vascularization is the process of tumor invasion (Fig. 1-4). Local tumor invasion results from local pressure of the tumor mass on normal tissues and the elaboration of substances such as type IV collagenase and heparinase that lead to enzymatic destruc-

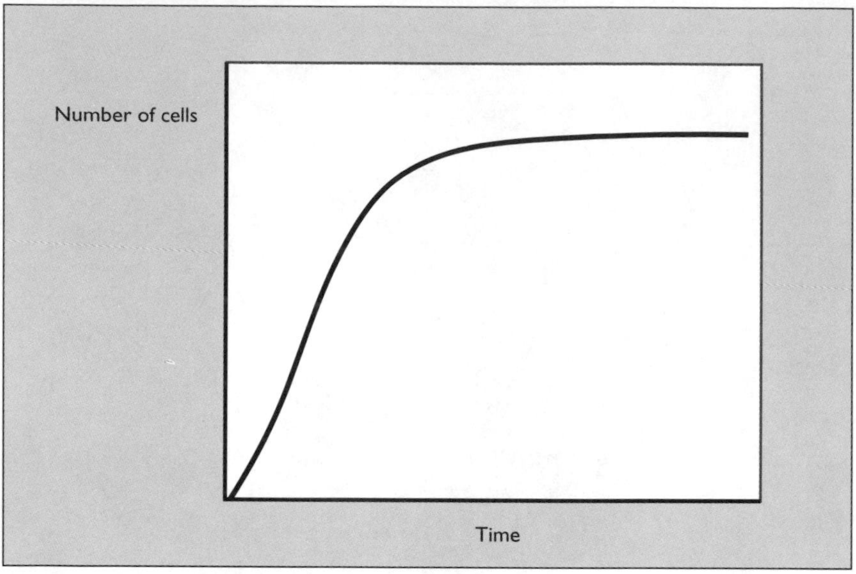

Figure 1-3 Tumor growth is characteristically depicted by a Gompertzian curve. An initial exponential phase of growth is followed by a plateau phase, when a "steady state" is reached; the rate of cell birth equals that of cellular death.

Table 1-1 Factors That Govern Tumor Growth

Promoting Tumor Growth	Inhibiting Tumor Growth
Anti-apoptotic	**Pro-apoptotic**
Overexpression of *bcl*-2	Wild-type p53
Overexpression of *bcl*-1	Bax
Pro-angiogenesis	**Anti-angiogenesis**
β-fibroblast growth factor	Naturally synthesized endostatin
Vascular endothelial growth factor	Naturally synthesized angiostatin
Cytokine and Steroid Soup in Extracellular Matrix	
Platelet-derived growth factor	Tumor necrosis factor
Interleukin 6	Interferon
Insulin-like growth factor	

tion. Small venules and lymphatic channels offer little resistance to the locally invasive tumor and provide the pathway for tumor cell entry into the circulation. Aggregates of tumor cells detach and embolize within the circulation. From work done in animal models, it is estimated that a 1-cm tumor sheds more than 1 million cells/24 h into the venous circulation. Most em-

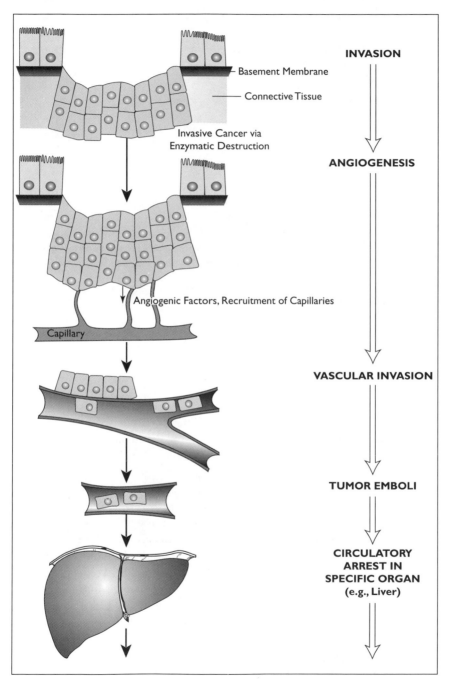

Figure 1-4 The process of metastasis.   *Continued.*

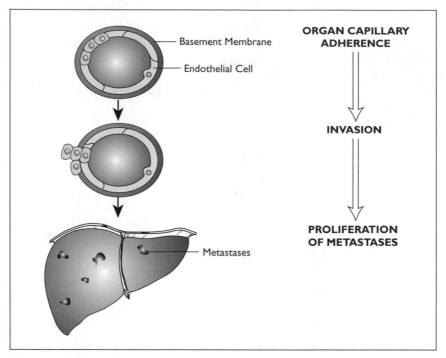

Figure 1-4 *Continued.*

bolized tumor cells are rapidly destroyed. The probability of a single cell or tumor aggregate surviving the "ride" within the circulation is less than one in a million. Those cells that survive the circulatory roller coaster ride adhere to the capillary beds of a distant organ. The adherence of the tumor cells or a tumor aggregate to the capillary bed is promoted by specific glycoproteins in the subendothelial basement membrane. Tumor cell elaboration of collagenase type IV is essential for its interaction with the subendothelial basement membrane and is also essential for invasion. Adherent tumor cells or aggregates now begin the process of extravasation through the capillary wall via enzymatic destruction (see Fig. 1-4). This satellite colony, *a metastasis*, begins the process of growth within the distant organ and the processes that follow—invasion, neovascularization, capillary bed invasion, and metastasis—begin anew.

Within any malignant tumor, certain cells are attracted to *specific metastatic sites* but not others. As the number of metastases increases, a metastatic nodule can give rise to other metastases. As shown in Table 1-2, the process of metastasis is not random and involves a complex interaction between the tumor and the host.

Table 1-2 Factors That Regulate the Metastatic Process

Facilitation of Metastatic Process	Inhibition of Metastasis
Tumor cell production of:	Tumor cell antigenicity
Growth factors and growth factor receptors	Tissue barriers
Angiogenic factors	Blood turbulence
Tumor cell motility	Tissue inhibitors of destructive
Tumor cell deformability	enzymes
Tumor cell invasiveness	Immunocompetent cells and their
Adherence molecules	products
Host facilitation of neovascularization	
Host paracrine and endocrine growth factors	
Platelets and platelet-derived products	
Host immunocompetent cells and their products	

Etiologic Agents Involved in Malignant Transformation

The etiologic agents involved in the multi-step process of malignant transformation are shown in Table 1-3. Viruses, environmental factors, and immunologic diseases are all etiologic factors. Within the United States, environmental and cultural habits account for most malignancies. Alcohol use and tobacco use combined account for nearly one third of the malignancies diagnosed within the U.S. Moreover, the incidence of melanoma has increased dramatically in this decade. Sun bathing and failure to use sunscreens accounts for this significant increase. Many of the drugs prescribed to treat a variety of inflammatory disorders or used to prevent the rejection of organ transplants can lead to malignancies. The prolonged use of alkylating agents such as melphalan, thiotepa, and chlorambucil have been linked to the development of acute nonlymphocytic leukemia (ANNL) that has a consistent chromosomal abnormality (discussed later in this chapter). Cyclosporine, which is commonly used to prevent rejection of solid organ transplants, can cause a lymphoproliferative disorder that may evolve into a malignant lymphoma. Phenacetin has been linked with both bladder and renal cell cancer; azathioprine has been linked to ANNL.

Patients with immunologic disorders, immunodeficiency disorders and diseases (e.g., systemic lupus erythematosus) that "turn on" the immune system, are predisposed to malignant lymphoma. Patients with ataxia-telangiectasia are predisposed to acute lymphoblastic leukemia (ALL), malignant lymphoma, and breast cancer. Patients with Wiskott-Aldrich syndrome and X-linked agammaglobulinemia are predisposed to ALL and malignant lymphoma.

Table 1-3 Etiologic Agents Involved in Malignant Transformation

Etiologic Agents	Cancer
Infectious Agents	
Viruses	
Cytomegalovirus	Kaposi sarcoma
Epstein-Barr virus	Burkitt lymphoma, lymphoblastic lymphoma, nasopharyngeal cancer
Human papilloma virus	Cervical cancer
HTLV-1	T-cell leukemia/lymphoma
HTLV-2	Hairy cell leukemia
Hepatitis B and C	Hepatocellular carcinoma
Herpes virus 8	Multiple myeloma
Parasites	
Schistosoma haematobium	Bladder cancer
Clonorchis sinensis	Pancreatic cancer, biliary cancer
Environmental Factors	
Chemicals	
Aromatic amines	Bladder cancer
Arsenic	Lung cancer
Asbestos	Lung cancer, mesothelioma
Benzene	Leukemia
Benzidine	Bladder cancer
Chromates	Lung cancer
Coal tar/pitch	Skin cancer, lung cancer, scrotum cancer
Magenta	Bladder cancer
Nickel	Lung cancer, cancer of the nasal sinuses
Vinyl chloride	Hepatocelllular carcinoma, angiosarcoma
Cultural habits	
Alcohol	Head and neck cancer, hepatocellular carcinoma
Sunbathing	Skin cancer
Tobacco (smoke)	Respiratory tract cancer, bladder cancer, pancreatic cancer
Tobacco (smokeless)	Oral cavity cancer
Drugs	
Analgesics with phenacetin	Kidney cancer, bladder cancer
Azathioprine	Leukemia
Chlorambucil	Leukemia
Cyclophosphamide	Leukemia
Cyclosporine	Lymphoma
Estrogens	Endometrial cancer, breast cancer (?)
Melphalan	Leukemia
Oral contraceptives	Liver cancer
Thiotepa	Leukemia

Table 1-3 Etiologic Agents Involved in Malignant Transformation—cont'd

Etiologic Agents	Cancer
Radiation	
Ionizing	Leukemia, breast cancer, lung cancer, bone cancer, sarcomas
Radon	Lung cancer
Ultraviolet	Skin cancer
Immunolgic factors	
Ataxia-telangiectasia	Leukemia, central nervous system cancer, gastric cancer
Rheumatoid arthritis	B-cell lymphoma
Sjögren syndrome	B-cell lymphoma
Systemic lupus erythematosus	B-cell lymphoma
Wiskott-Aldrich syndrome	Leukemia, lymphoma
X-linked agammaglobulinemia	Leukemia, lymphoma

Patients with acquired immunodeficiency syndrome (AIDS) are predisposed to a variety of cancers including Kaposi sarcoma, malignant lymphoma, and rectal and oropharyngeal cancers. Patients with systemic lupus erythematosus, rheumatoid arthritis, and Sjögren syndrome are predisposed to malignant lymphoma.

The Molecular Biology of Malignant Transformation and Cancer Genetics

Cancer is a genetic disease. It is genetic because mutational events in three classes of cellular genes—*oncogenes, tumor suppressor genes,* and *DNA repair genes*—lead to cancer. Although inherited mutations, environmental factors, and dietary factors all influence the process of malignant transformation, the prevailing view is that cancers arise from the accumulation of multiple mutations in a single cell. The study of oncogenes carried out by acute transforming retroviruses facilitated the identification of many human genes with critical roles in cellular growth and differentiation (1).

Oncogenes

The *ras* family of genes encodes for a guanine nucleotide-binding protein with a molecular weight of 21,000 kD (p21). The ras proteins are involved in the signal transduction of activated growth and/or differentiation receptors to downstream protein kinases. The *ras* family includes K-*ras*, N-*ras*, and H-*ras*. The codon 12 of K-*ras* is a frequent target of point mutations, particularly in colorectal cancer, pancreatic cancer, and adenocarcinoma of the lung. Patients with adenocarcinoma of the lung whose tumors harbor a mutant K-*ras* gene have a poorer prognosis than those whose tumors do not harbor this mutation.

The *myc* genes, *myc*, N-*myc*, and L-*myc*, function in the regulation of cellular growth. The myc proteins, following dimerization with a protein called Max, function as transcriptional factors by binding to specific DNA sequences. Activation of *myc* genes can occur as a result of chromosomal translocations, as for example in malignant B-cell lymphomas. In these lymphomas, the heavy-chain immunoglobulin sequences on chromosome 14 are fused with the sequence for the *myc* gene on chromosome 8. The *myc* gene locus can be activated when the kappa light-chain sequences on chromosome 2 or the lambda light-chain sequence on chromosome 22 are translocated to chromosome 8. Activation of *myc* has also been reported in small cell lung cancer (*myc*, L-*myc*, and N-*myc*) and neuroblastoma (N-*myc*). Patients with limited-stage neuroblastoma and N-*myc* amplification have a poorer prognosis than patients with no N-*myc* amplification.

The *neu* gene family (*Her-2/neu* or c-*erb*-b2) is located on the long arm of chromosome 17 (17q) and encodes for a phosphoprotein that is very similar to the epidermal growth factor receptor. To date, the specific peptide ligand for the *neu* gene receptor has not been discovered. Overexpression of the *neu* gene has prognostic importance in women with node-negative breast cancer. Women with stage I breast cancer whose cancer overexpresses the *neu* gene have a poorer prognosis than do patients with no overexpression of *neu*. Recently, a murine monoclonal antibody directed against the *neu* receptor has been approved by the FDA and is quite useful in the treatment of women with stage IV breast cancer who have significant overexpression of the *neu* gene.

The *bcl*-2 gene belongs to a superfamily of genes that regulate programmed cell death or apoptosis. The *bcl*-2 gene is but one of several death antagonist/agonist genes. The *bcl*-2 gene is activated in malignant B-cell lymphomas by a chromosomal translocation in which the immunoglobulin heavy-chain sequence on chromosome 14 is translocated to the *bcl*-2 sequence on the long arm of chromosome 18. This translocation results in the overexpression of *bcl*-2 mRNA and their encoded proteins. When *bcl*-2 is overexpressed, it encodes for the *bcl*-2 protein that then forms heterodimers with death promoting proteins (Bid, Bad, and Bax) and in turn inhibits apoptosis. Overexpression of *bcl*-2 leads to a relative overabundance of this antiapoptotic protein. Overexpression of *bcl*-2 is common in B-cell lymphomas as well as in breast cancer. It appears that overexpression of *bcl*-2 is not necessarily a poor prognostic factor in patients with malignant lymphomas, and patients with *bcl*-2 overexpression tend to have a better prognosis than those who do not. Similarly, in women with breast cancer, those who have *bcl*-2 overexpression tend to have a better overall prognosis than those who do not.

Tumor Suppressor Genes

The ability of certain classes of cellular genes to suppress tumorigenicity in vitro via the transfer of intact genetic material confirms the presence of a class of genes that have important regulatory functions in cellular growth (Table 1-4).

The retinoblastoma gene (*RB* gene) is located on the long arm of chromosome 13, band 14 (13q14), and encodes for a protein that has a molecular weight of 105,000 kD (p105-RB). The retinoblastoma protein is phosphorylated and hypophosphorylated during the cell cycle; when hypophosphorylated, it complexes with other proteins (E2F and DP), which regulate the transcription of several genes, including DNA polymerase, thymidine kinase, and dihydrofolate reductase (Fig. 1-5). Kudson's analysis of the inheritance patterns and age-specific incidence of retinoblastoma led him to propose that two mutagenic events ("two hits") were required for the development of retinoblastoma, the two hit hypothesis. The two hit hypothesis acknowledges that children with retinoblastoma carry an inherited (germline) mutation in one of the retinoblastoma alleles and that a second somatic mutation in the other alleles triggers retinoblastoma. Molecular studies in patients with retinoblastoma have confirmed the Kudson two hit hypothesis by demonstrating allelic loss (Fig. 1-6). Somatic mutations of the *RB* gene have been shown in small cell lung cancer, and breast, bladder, and prostate cancers.

The p53 gene on the short arm of chromosome 17 encodes for a transcriptional regulatory protein that controls the cell's ability to synthesize DNA at the G_1/S checkpoint of the cell cycle. The p53 gene has been dubbed "the guardian of the genome" because of its ability to arrest cellular growth in the G_1 phase in response to DNA damage and either to repair the damage before DNA synthesis or to lead to programmed cell death, apoptosis. The p53 gene accomplishes this by allowing transcription of p21, which leads to adenyl-

Table I-4 Tumor Suppressor Genes

Gene	Chromosome
Retinoblastoma (*RB*)	13q14
p53	17p
p73	1p
APC	5q21
NFI	17q
WTI	11p13
BRCAI (?)	17q21
BRCA2 (?)	13q
MSH2	2p
MLHI	3p
RET	10q11.2

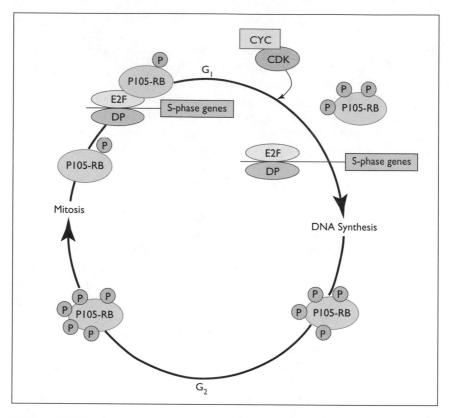

Figure 1-5 The normal function of the retinoblastoma protein. The degree of phosphorylation regulates the function of the retinoblastoma protein. The retinoblastoma protein is hypophosphorylated during the G_1 phase of the cell cycle, and the degree of phosphorylation of the retinoblastoma protein increases just before the S phase (DNA synthetic phase). As the retinoblastoma protein is phosphorylated, it uncomplexes from the E2F and the DP proteins, which in turn regulate several genes involved in DNA synthesis. The hypophosphorylated form of the retinoblastoma protein complexes with E2F and DP proteins. The E2F and DP proteins can then no longer participate in DNA synthesis, and therefore, no DNA synthesis occurs.

cyclin–induced cell cycle arrest. Thus, p53 *inactivation* allows for genomic instability. Inherited mutations of a single copy of the p53 gene cause the *Li-Fraumeni syndrome*. Persons with this syndrome are at high risk for soft tissue sarcomas, osteosarcomas, central nervous system (CNS) malignancies, leukemias, and breast cancer. As previously mentioned for the *RB* gene, a second somatic mutation of the p53 allele must take place for a malignancy to develop. It has become increasingly clear that p53 mutations are quite common in human malignancies and may represent a final common pathway in malig-

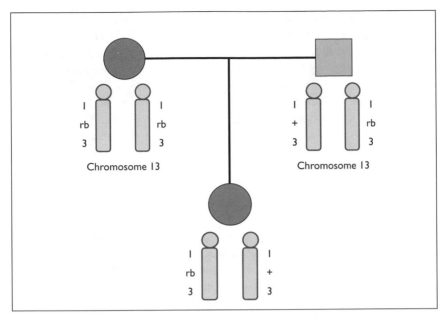

Figure 1-6 The inheritance of a predisposition to retinoblastoma is shown in this family. The normal retinoblastoma gene is depicted as *rb*. The father developed a somatic mutation at the *rb* locus, which is depicted as +. The affected daughter has a germline mutation that she inherited from her father. She is now predisposed to retinoblastoma. A second somatic mutation (second hit) at the normal *rb* allele will lead to retinoblastoma.

nant transformation. Point mutations of p53 have been reported in lung, colorectal, breast, bladder, and CNS cancers.

Another tumor suppressor gene, p73, has been discovered and has been mapped to the tip of the short arm of chromosome 1. The p73 gene also mediates p21 adenyl-cyclin cell cycle arrest at the G_1 checkpoint. Mutations of p73 may be implicated in neuroblastoma and breast and gastric cancers.

The adenomatous polyposis coli tumor suppressor gene (*APC* gene) is located on the long arm of chromosome 5 (5q21) and is deleted in persons with *familial adenomatous polyposis (FAP), or Gardner syndrome*. While germline mutations of the *APC* gene are responsible for FAP, somatic mutations of this gene may be critically important in the pathogenesis of colorectal adenomata and colorectal cancer (see Fig. 1-1). The function of the *APC* gene is as yet unknown.

The neurofibromatosis type I tumor suppressor gene (*NFI*) is located in the pericentromeric region of the long arm of chromosome 17 (17q). Although mutations of this gene are believed to be present in all patients with von Recklinghausen's neurofibromatosis (neurofibromas, café au lait spots, increased risk of pheochromocytomas, schwannomas, neurofibrosarcomas, and CNS tumors), germline mutations have been identified in only 15% to 20% of patients with von Recklinghausen's neurofibromatosis. The gene product of *NFI* is a protein called *neurofibromin*, which is very similar to GTPase-activating proteins involved in signal transduction. Somatic mutations of *NFI* have been reported in colorectal cancer, melanoma, neuroblastoma, and in the bone marrow specimens of patients with myelodysplasia.

The Wilms tumor suppressor gene (*WT1*) is located on the short arm of chromosome 11 (11p13). The gene products of *WT1* are a protein or proteins that function as transcriptional regulatory proteins. The inactivation of the *WT1* gene accounts for some but not all cases of Wilms tumor, and allelic loss and/or mutations involving other regions of 11p have been recently identified.

Within the past 2 years, two breast cancer genes have been identified: *BRCA1* and *BRCA2*. The *BRCA1* gene is located on the long arm of chromosome 17 (17q21) and when mutated is responsible for "genetic" or familial breast cancer. Patients with familial breast cancer have a strong family history of breast cancer that is inherited as an autosomal dominant; the average age of onset is less than 45 years. Persons with germline *BRCA1* mutations have a greater than 65% risk of developing breast cancer in their lifetimes. Mutations of *BRCA1* also increase the risk of ovarian cancer. Some estimates are that 1 of every 200 women in the United States harbors a germline mutation in *BRCA1*. Moreover, U.S. women of Ashkenazi Jewish heritage have a higher incidence of germline mutations in *BRCA1* (3 to 4 per 100 women). The protein products of *BRCA1* have been recently identified and appear to function as nuclear regulatory proteins. Men with germline mutations of *BRCA1* appear to be at increased risk for prostate cancer.

The *BRCA2* gene has recently been cloned and is localized to the long arm of chromosome 13. Women with germline mutations of *BRCA2* are at increased risk for breast cancer. The function and protein product of *BRCA2* is unknown.

Hereditary nonpolyposis colorectal cancer (HNPCC) is an inherited disease in which a germline mutation predisposes persons to colorectal cancer. There are four criteria needed to establish a diagnosis of HNPCC: (1) absence of familial polyposis; (2) family history of colorectal cancer in at least three relatives and of whom at least one is a first-degree relative; (3) family history of colorectal cancer affecting two or more generations; and (4) onset of the colorectal cancer occurs at less than 50 years old. Two types of HNPCC have been described. HNPCC-Lynch-I is solely colorectal cancer; Lynch-II is colorectal cancer associated with endometrial, bladder, or hepatobiliary cancer. The genes involved in HNPCC have been localized to chromosomes 2p and 3p and are *MSH2* (2p) and *MLH1* (3p). Both of these genes are involved in DNA repair.

Multiple endocrine neoplasia (MEN) is an inherited disease in which persons are predisposed to neoplasms of the pituitary, pancreas, or parathyroid (MEN 1) or to medullary thyroid carcinoma, pheochromocytoma, and parathyroid adenomas (MEN 2). MEN 2 is further divided into MEN 2A and MEN 2B; MEN 2B is associated with mucosal neuromas. The chromosomal abnormality that is linked to both MEN 2A and MEN 2B are mutations of the *RET* gene, which is located on the long arm of chromosome 10 (10q11.2). Germline mutations of the *RET* gene predispose persons to MEN 2A or 2B.

Cancer Genetics

As previously stated, cancer is a genetic disease. Germline or acquired somatic genetic mutations initiate the neoplastic process. Nonrandom chromosomal abnormalities are associated with specific cancers (Table 1-5). Chronic myelogenous leukemia (CML) and acute promyelocytic leukemia (APL) are prototypic models of specific genetic mutations in early hematopoietic progenitor cells that in turn lead to specific disease processes. In CML, the translocation of a portion of the long arm of chromosome 9 to chromosome 22 leads to the production of a mutant fusion protein that exhibits increased tyrosine kinase activity, which in turn causes clonal proliferation of the cells bearing this mutation. In APL, the *PML* gene on chromosome 15 is translocated and fuses with the retinoic acid receptor gene alpha (*rar-α*) on chromosome 17. The resultant chimeric proteins from the fused *PML/rar-α* transcript may block the ability of retinoic acid to regulate the process of myeloid cell differentiation. Pharmacologic doses of all-*trans*-retinoic acid down regulate the expression of these chimeric proteins and thus allow normal differentiation. The 14;18 translocation in B-cell non-Hodgkin lymphoma (NHL) leads to the overexpression of the *bcl*-2 gene. The overexpression of *bcl*-2 is important in the pathogenesis of B-cell NHL and prevents apoptosis. Chemotherapeutics used in the treatment of NHL may work by down-regulating *bcl*-2 overexpression and allow for the normal apoptotic pathways to take place.

In addition to the syndromes that we have already discussed in this chapter, several other important albeit rare hereditary syndromes predispose adults and children to malignancies (Tables 1-6 and 1-7). Many of the mutated genes associated with these hereditary syndromes have been cloned and identified. Genetic testing is already available that can identify mutations within the *BRCA1* locus. During the ensuing decade, a wide variety of genetic testing will be available to identify high-risk populations. However, genetic testing cannot be conducted indiscriminately. A detailed family history is fundamental in assessing the probability of a hereditary cancer syndrome. Table 1-8 shows the

Table 1-5 Chromosomal Abnormalities Associated with Neoplasms

Neoplasm	Genes	Chromosomal Abnormalities
Acute myeloid leukemia		
with maturation		t(8;21)
with basophilia	PEK/CAN	t(6;9)
Acute myelomonocytic leukemia		
with eosinophilia		inv. 16
Acute monocytic leukemia		11q–
Acute lymphoblastic leukemia		t(4;11), also t(9;22)
Acute promyelocytic leukemia	rar-α/PML	t(15;17)
Chronic lymphoblastic leukemia		+12
Chronic myeloid leukemia	ABL/BCR	t(9;22)
Malignant lymphomas		
Burkitt lymphoma	myc/IgH	t(8;14), also t(8;22) and t(2;8)
Non-Hodgkin lymphoma		
B cell	Igκ/myc	t(2;8)
	/IgH	t(2;14)
	myc/IgH	t(8;14)
	IgH/bcl-2	t(14;18)
	IgH/bcl-3	t(14;19)
Mantle zone		t(14;11q13)
MALT	IgH/bcl-10	t(11;14)
T cell	Tcrβ/TAL2	t(7;19)
	Tcrβ/TAN	t(7;9)
	Tcrβ/	t(7;11)
	Tcrβ/LYL1	t(7;19)
Solid tumors		
Meningiomas		22q–
Salivary gland (mixed)		t(3;8), also t(9;12)
Colonic polyps		5p–
Small cell lung cancer		3p–
Renal cell cancer		3p–
Uterine cancer		1p–
Prostate cancer		7q–, also 10q–
Bladder cancer		–9 also –11 and –15
Ovarian cancer		t(6;14)
Colon cancer		17q– also 18q–
Testis cancer		inv.12
Malignant melanoma		6q–, also inv.6
Mesothelioma		3p–
Liposarcoma		t(12;16)
Synovial sarcoma		t(x;18)
Rhabdomyosarcoma		t(2;13)
Chondrosarcoma		t(9;22)
Ewing sarcoma		t(11;22)
Retinoblastoma	RB1	13q–
Wilm tumor	WT1	11p–
Neuroblastoma	NF1	1p–

MALT = mucosa-associated lymphoid tissue.

Table 1-6 Hereditary Cancer Syndromes in Adults

Syndrome	Mode of Inheritance	Gene/ Chromosome	Cancer
Familial breast cancer	Dominant	BRCA1/17q	Breast, ovary
	Dominant	BRCA2/13q	Breast
Li-Fraumeni	Dominant	p53/17p	Breast, CNS, adrenal
Familial prostate cancer	Dominant		Prostate
Cowden disease	Dominant		Breast, hamartomas
Adenomatous polyposis coli (Gardner syndrome)	Dominant	APC/5q	Colon
Hereditary nonpolyposis colorectal cancer			
Type I	Dominant	MLH1/3p	Colon
Type II	Dominant	MSH2/2p	Colon, endometrial
Turcot syndrome	Recessive		Polyposis, CNS
Multiple endocrine neoplasia (MEN)			
Type I	Dominant	/11q	Pancreatic islet cell
Type 2	Dominant	RET/10	Medullary, thyroid
Dysplastic nevus syndrome	Dominant	/1p	Melanoma, meningioma
Gorlin syndrome	Dominant	/9q	Basal cell
Neurofibromatosis			
Type I	Dominant	NF1/17q	Sarcomas, optic gliomas, pheochromocytomas
Type 2	Dominant	Merlin/22q	Sarcomas, gliomas
von-Hippel-Lindau disease	Dominant	VHL /3p	Renal cell, pheochromo-cytomas
Familial renal cancer	Dominant	VHL ?/3p	Renal
Familial lymphoproliferative			Lymphomas

Table 1-7 Hereditary Cancer Syndromes in Children

Syndrome	Mode of Inheritance	Gene/ Chromosome	Cancer
Retinoblastoma	Dominant	RB1/13q	Retinoblastoma
Wilm tumor	Dominant	WT1/11p	Wilm tumor
Fanconi syndrome	Recessive	FACC/	Leukemia
			Esophageal
Ataxia-telangiectasia	Recessive	/11q	Leukemia
			Lymphoma
			Ovarian
Bloom syndrome	Recessive	/15	Leukemia
			Esophageal
			Head and neck
			Wilm tumor
Xeroderma pigmentosum	Recessive	RAD2/	Skin, melanoma
X-linked lymphoprolifera-tive syndrome	Recessive	/Xq	Lymphoma, chronic lymphatic leukemia

lifetime risk of selected cancers based on family history. As shown in this table, risk is dependent on the relative (e.g., first-, second-, or third-degree) who developed the cancer in question and on the age of that relative when the cancer first developed. It would be imprudent to look for a *BRCA1* mutation in a woman who has only a second- or third-degree relative with breast cancer. As demonstrated in Table 1-8, in a woman with a second- or third-degree relative with breast cancer, the overall risk is 1.4. With such a low risk, genetic breast cancer and specifically a *BRCA1* mutation are unlikely. In contrast, a *BRCA1* mutation is much more likely in a woman who has a family history of a mother and sister who developed bilateral breast cancer at less than 49 years of age.

If a proband is suspected of having a hereditary cancer syndrome, genetic counseling should be undertaken before any definitive testing is done. The patient and his or her family require a frank and open discussion of what it means to be a carrier of a hereditary cancer syndrome and of what steps can be taken to reduce risk. Once the patient and his or her family understand the risks and benefits of genetic testing, definitive testing can be carried out with further counseling after the results are known. Genetic counselors are prepared to deal with the depression and guilt felt by the carriers and with the "survivor's guilt" felt by the noncarriers.

Identification of high-risk cancer populations and risk reduction will be increasingly important in the decades to come. Although some may consider genetic testing to be futile because of the assumption that "nothing can be done" to prevent inherited cancer syndromes anyway, the truth is that physicians and patients *will* behave differently when high-risk individuals are identified through genetic testing. If a physician knows that a patient carries a *BRCA1* or *BRCA2* mutation, a dominant breast lump will be excised rather than watched. Pleiotropic calcifications on mammography will be biopsied rather than observed. Moreover, recent studies have shown that prophylactic mastectomy lowers the risk of breast cancer in women who carry *BRCA1* mutations. Clearly, the hope is that other means of risk reduction will be available in the near future.

Risk Reduction

Once high-risk populations have been identified, methods of reducing risk need to be employed (Case 1-1, p 20). There are currently four ongoing chemoprevention trials, with the collective end point being a reduction in cancer incidence. A large trial attempting to reduce the incidence of breast cancer in women at risk compared tamoxifen with placebo and showed a 45% risk reduction in breast cancer with the use of tamoxifen, 20 mg/d for 5 years (2). Premenopausal women at risk for breast cancer should be treated with tamoxifen.

Table 1-8 Lifetime Risk of Selected Cancers in Probands with a Family History

Cancer	Risk (1 = normal)
Breast cancer	
Mother, sister (any age)	2–4
Sister <49 yr	3.6–5
Sister bilateral <40 yr	11
Mother and sister bilateral <49 yr	39
Second- or third-degree relative	1.3–1.4
Colon cancer	
Mother, father, siblings	3–7
First-degree relative <60 yr with polyp	3.6
First-degree relative >70 yr with polyp	1.4
Family history of colon cancer with a polyp in proband	3
Ovarian cancer	
First-degree relative	4
Prostate cancer	
First-degree relative	2–5
Melanoma	
First-degree relative	2.7

Table 1-9 Risk Reduction for Individuals with Hereditary Cancer Syndromes

Syndrome	Recommendations
Familial breast cancer	Intense surveillance, prophylactic mastectomy, tamoxifen
Adenomatous polyposis coli	Colectomy
Hereditary nonpolyposis colorectal cancer	Colectomy, aspirin, or nonsteroidal anti-inflammatories
Multiple endocrine neoplasia, type II	Thyroidectomy
Dysplastic nevus syndrome	Photographic surveillance/excision of suspicious lesions

Postmenopausal women at risk for breast cancer should be encouraged to enroll in a clinical trial comparing tamoxifen with raloxifene. Similar trials are ongoing in men at risk for prostate cancer (finasteride compared with placebo), colon cancer (aspirin compared with placebo), and lung cancer (cis-retinoic acid compared with placebo). In these trials, at-risk populations have been identified based on age or the presence of underlying premalignant disease (e.g., lobular carcinoma in situ, polyps) or a history of a surgically cured malignancy (e.g., lung cancer). Definitive recommendations as to the usefulness of any chemopreventative agent cannot be made at this time; however, both aspirin and non-steroidal anti-inflammatory drugs have been shown to decrease the incidence of colon cancer in patients with colonic polyps. Recommendations for attempts to reduce cancer risk in individuals with hereditary cancer syndromes are shown in Table 1-9.

Case 1-1

A 49-year-old white nurse sees her primary care physician to have her risk of breast cancer evaluated. Her visit has been prompted by the recent diagnosis of ovarian cancer in a maternal aunt. The patient is very concerned about reducing her risk. She has a family history of one of four maternal aunts developing breast cancer at age 50 years and of two of four maternal aunts developing ovarian cancer between the ages of 60 and 70 years. The daughter of one of the maternal aunts with ovarian cancer was diagnosed with breast cancer at age 45 years. The patient's mother, who is 73 years old, is alive and well. There is no family history of cancer on her father's side. Since being diagnosed as menopausal 1 year ago, she has been using hormone replacement therapy and is anxious about continuing it. She exercises religiously 5 to 6 days per week and eats a low-fat diet. Menarche was at age 12 years and up until age 47 years her periods were regular, occurring once every 27 to 28 days. She used birth control pills from age 21 to 24 years. She has been pregnant three times and has a son (age 25 years) and two daughters (ages 17 and 12), who are in good health. Two years ago she had a fibroadenoma removed from her right breast.

The only abnormal physical finding is the presence of fibrocystic disease in the right breast and a healed surgical scar. The remainder of the physical examation is unremarkable.

The familial history of breast and ovarian cancer raise the possibility of genetic breast or ovarian cancer and a BRCA1 mutation (see Table 1.6).

The patient is advised that genetic testing may be appropriate and is counseled regarding the risks and potential benefits. She is referred to a geneticist and has genetic counseling before any testing is begun.

The testing demonstrates that she is a BRCA1 carrier, and she returns for further recommendations.

She is advised to discontinue hormone replacement therapy, and the risks and benefits of a prophylactic mastectomy are reviewed. She makes the decision to have prophylactic oophorectomy to diminish her risk for ovarian cancer, which is 30% lifetime. She chooses at the same time to undergo a bilateral mastectomy and reconstruction to diminish her risk of breast cancer, which is 65% lifetime.

REFERENCES

1. **Fearon ER.** Oncogenes and tumor suppressor genes. In: Abeloff MD, Armitage JO, Lichter AS, Niederhuber JE, eds. Clinical Oncology. New York: Churchill Livingstone; 1995:11-40.

2. **Fisher B, Costatino JP, Wickerham DL, et al.** Tamoxifen for prevention of breast cancer: report of the National Surgical Adjuvant Breast and Bowel Project P-1 Study. J Natl Cancer Inst. 1998;90:1371-88.

Chapter 2

Establishing a Diagnosis

History and Physical Examination

The primary care physician is generally the first member of the medical team to establish a diagnosis of malignancy. The basis of establishing a diagnosis is a complete and thorough history and physical examination (H&P). The time-held adage that 80% of diagnoses are based on the H&P is still true today, even in the current age of techno-medicine.

A review of systems is important. Aspects of the history that must be elicited in detail include symptoms such as mouth soreness, difficulty in mastication, sore throat, ear pain, loose teeth or ill fitting dentures, hoarseness, unexplained oropharyngeal pain, unexplained nasal stuffiness, nasal bleeding, shortness of breath, cough, chest pain or pressure, hemoptysis, change in bowel habits, abdominal pain or cramping, abdominal distension, early satiety, incomplete rectal evacuation, melena, or hematochezia, hematuria, unexplained fever, flank or back pain, weight loss, enlarged lymph nodes, and pain on weight bearing. The history should also elicit information regarding the duration and intensity of any such symptoms, as well as what, if anything, brings about relief of the symptoms. The review of systems is not a mere exercise in futility but rather a thorough, careful, detailed review of the patient's history by inquiring for salient symptoms associated with each anatomic region. It is a search for symptoms that may have escaped notice during the history taking for the present illness that has prompted the patient's visit.

The past medical history is obviously likewise important and should include queries as to the exposure to human immunodeficiency virus, Epstein-Barr virus, and hepatitis B and C. A complete history of prior malignancies and their treatment may shed light on the current symptoms. Furthermore, as discussed in Chapter 1, a detailed family history is essential in determining the risk of malignancy. The patient's social history is relevant, because it yields information regarding occupational exposure to environmental causes of malignancy as well as regarding tobacco and alcohol consumption.

The physical examination is crucial, and specific anatomic areas deserve particular attention. A detailed evaluation of the head and neck with close attention to the oropharynx, tongue, and thyroid is mandatory. In examining the oropharynx, the physician should have the patient lean slightly forward and relax the shoulders, neck, and chin. The gums should be examined and the tongue and its undersurface should be inspected, as well as the hard and soft palates. The presence of induration, edema, erythema, or ulceration should be noted. Typically, a carcinoma in the oral cavity is a shallow ulcer with prominent lateral borders. The tongue and floor of the mouth should be palpated with a gloved finger (this will elicit a gag reflex so it should be done last). Because several cancers in these areas are submucosal, they may not be visually detected and palpation of a firm area may be the only sign of pathology. Deep-seated ear pain in the absence of any visible abnormality may be a symptom of an oropharyngeal cancer. Primary care physicians should be familiar with the normal palpable landmarks of the anatomy of the neck: the sternocleidomastoid muscles, the carotid bulb, the cartilaginous landmarks of the larynx, and the submandibular glands.

A thorough examination of lymph node–bearing regions, including the cervical, supraclavicular, axillary, epitrochlear, inguinal, and femoral nodal regions, is mandatory. Painless lymph nodal enlargement is characteristic of a neoplastic process. Two of every three patients with non-Hodgkin lymphoma present with a chief symptom of painless enlarged lymph nodes. The presence of an enlarged lymph node (≥1 cm) does not necessarily imply malignancy or lymphoma. In children and adults, palpable inguinal lymph nodes 0.5 to 2 cm in size may be found during a routine physical examination; these nodes are palpable and enlarged because of repeated inflammatory stimuli. In children, enlarged nodes in the cervical or axillary region may be a consequence of past infections. It is important to elicit a history of any recent travel, occupational exposure, or exposure to infectious agents or their vectors during recreational activities. The causes of lymphadenopathy are listed in Table 2-1. In adults, enlarged lymph nodes (>1 cm) in regions other the inguinal region constitute a pathologic finding and require diagnostic work-up unless an underlying cause is known. With in-

Table 2-1 The Causes of Lymphadenopathy

Infectious
Viral
  Adenovirus
  Cytomegalovirus
  Epstein-Barr virus
  Hepatitis virus
  Human immunodeficiency virus
  Lymphogranuloma venereum
  Rubella
  Rubeola
  Trachoma
Rickettsial
  Q fever
  Rocky Mountain spotted fever
Protozoan
  Amebiasis
  Cat-scratch fever
  Toxoplasmosis
Bacterial
  Anthrax
  Brucellosis
  Chancroid
  Diphtheria
  Leprosy
  Listeriosis
  Mycobacterium tuberculosis
  Atypical *Mycobacterium*
  Plague
  Rat bite fever
  Tularemia
Fungal
  Blastomycosis
  Coccidiomycosis
  Histoplasmosis
  Ringworm
  Sporotrichiosis
Spirochetal
  Leptospirosis
  Syphilis

Immunologic
  Carbamazepine
  Dilantin
  Graft-versus-host disease
  Hemolytic anemia
  Rheumatoid arthritis
  Serum sickness
  Systemic lupus erythematosus

Neoplastic
  Acute leukemias
  Chronic lymphatic leukemia
  Chronic myelogenous leukemia
  Hodgkin disease
  Metastatic carcinomas or sarcomas
  Myelosclerosis
  Non-Hodgkin lymphoma

Other
  Addison disease
  Amyloidosis
  Chronic granulomatous disease
  Dermatopathic lymphadenitis
  Follicular hyperplasia
  Gaucher disease
  Mucocutaneous lymph node syndrome
  Multifocal Langerhans cell (eosinophilic)
    granulomatosis
  Necrotizing lymphadenitis
  Neiman-Pick disease
  Sarcoid
  Silicone
  Sinus histiocytosis
  Thyrotoxicosis
  Vaccina

fection, involved lymph nodes are usually asymmetrically enlarged, tender, and matted together; the overlying skin may be erythematous. *With metastatic cancer, lymph nodes are usually hard and fixed to the underlying tissues. Lymph nodal involvement by lymphoma tends to cause firm, nontender, and usually matted lymph nodes.* In adults, a biopsy should be performed on a newly enlarged lymph node (>1 cm) if an underlying cause cannot be determined. The presence of lymphadenopathy of any size in the epitrochlear, supraclavicular, and femoral regions is *always pathologic and always requires a biopsy.*

A thorough examination of the chest and lungs is required. One needs to look at the the pattern of respirations and at the chest. Is the breathing labored? Does the patient have fullness in the neck and conjunctival sufflation, which indicates a superior vena cava (SVC) syndrome? Are there prominent chest wall veins that may be indicative of a chronic SVC syndrome? Is there any evidence of localized wheezing or rhonchi, rales or pleural friction rubs, dullness, "e to a" change, or egophony? Although any of these findings is not necessarily indicative of malignancy, one should try to discover the cause. If wheezing, rhonchi, and rales are associated with a fever, it may be reasonable to conclude that the patient has a pulmonary infection and to administer the appropriate treatment, with the expectation that the patient should improve within 2 weeks. However, the continued presence of such findings requires a prompt investigation, because the patient may in fact have a postobstructive pneumonia secondary to an intraluminal bronchial mass or a bronchoalveolar carcinoma. In contrast, the presence of dullness with absent breath sounds and/or pleural friction rubs should be investigated promptly with chest radiography. The physician needs to keep in mind that patients with superior sulcus tumors rarely present with symptoms of a cough but rather with dull upper chest and arm pain caused by early infiltration of the brachial plexus.

When examining the abdomen, the physician should look for the presence of ascites, hepatic or splenic enlargement, and abdominal masses and/or midline fullness. Although the presence of an enlarged liver or spleen is pathologic, it does not necessarily indicate malignancy. The presence and location of an abdominal mass or abdominal fullness may provide clues as to the site of origin. A right lower quadrant mass may reflect a cecal cancer. Midline upper quadrant fullness usually reflects retroperitoneal adenopathy and/or masses and may indicate lymphoma, retroperitoneal sarcomas, or metastases to retroperitoneal lymph nodes. Metastases to the peritoneum cause the presence of an omental cake (Fig. 2-1), which is an upper quadrant mass extending both to the right and left. Omental cakes are finely nodular on palpation and in women usually reflect metastases from ovarian cancer or a primary peritoneal malignancy. The rectal examination should include inspection of the perirectal skin as well as a digital examination of the rectum and, in men, the prostate. In examining the perirectal skin, the physician should look for the presence of "warts," which are small exophytic tumors (condyloma acuminata); reddened or indurated skin patches (anal intraepithelial neoplasia, Bowen disease); or encrusted or ulcerated patches (Paget disease). Bowen disease, which was at one time rare, has become increasingly more common, especially among persons with human immunodeficiency virus (HIV). Anal Paget disease usually is associated with an underlying anal cancer. The rectal

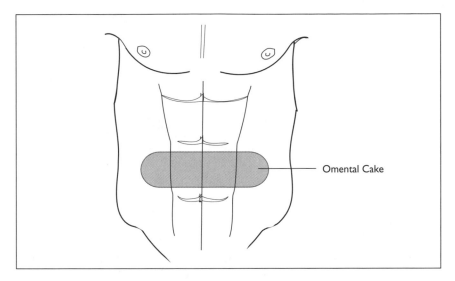

Omental Cake

Figure 2-1 On physical examination, the typical location of an "omental cake."

digital examination is performed to detect masses in the anal or rectal area. A mass in this area indicates cancer until proven otherwise. The examiner should also watch for a rectal shelf, a mass or fullness external to the rectum, that is reflective of peritoneal metastases. In men, the rectal examination affords an opportunity to examine the prostate for signs of enlargement, nodularity, or masses. Upon completion of the rectal digital examination, the stool on the glove tip should be examined for the presence of occult blood.

In women, a careful examination of the breasts is an integral part of the physical examination. The breasts should be observed with the woman sitting up with her hands on her waist and then with her hands behind her head. The physician should watch for bulges, dimpling, and peau d'orange. With the woman in the supine position, the physician should then palpate the breasts. My preferred method is to place my hand over the top of the breast just below the clavicle and palpate by running three fingers across the breast linearly. The area of the breast just below is also palpated in a similar manner, and one continues in a "staircase" manner as shown in Figure 2-2*A*. This is in contrast to the concentric circular method of palpation shown in Figure 2-2*B*. A dominant mass is one that stands out from the otherwise "normal" lumpy breast tissue. A careful examination of the extremities and flanks should include palpation for any masses.

The last parts of the physical examination—the cardiac and neurologic examinations—should be conducted with great care. In particular, a detailed neurologic examination should include a cranial nerve examination and assessment of deep tendon reflexes, pathologic reflexes, muscle strength, gait, propriocep-

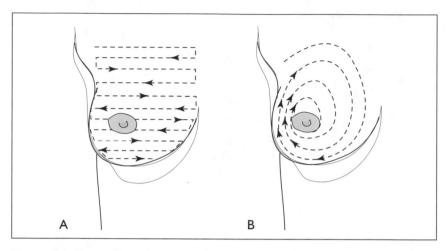

Figure 2-2 Two methods for examining the breast. The usual method involves examination of the breast by palpation along concentric circles (*B*). An alternative method is to palpate in a linear ("staircase") manner (*A*). In the author's experience, this method is easier and more thorough.

tive sense, memory, and the patient's ability to perform simple calculations. The symptoms of primary brain tumors are insidious. Headaches and symptoms of increased intracranial pressure are often late findings. The early manifestations of brain tumors may be nothing more than difficulty concentrating and making errors in performing simple calculations.

As previously stated, the history and physical examination should provide a tentative diagnosis 80% of the time, and any abnormal physical findings should prompt additional testing.

Obtaining a Tissue Diagnosis

Obtaining a tissue diagnosis is central to establishing a diagnosis of malignancy and key to cancer staging and management.

Fine-Needle Aspiration

Fine-needle aspiration (FNA) of a mass in the breast, thyroid, or lung often establishes a diagnosis of malignancy. A solitary palpable thyroid nodule should first be evaluated with a Tc-99m thyroid scan to determine if it is a "hot" nodule, which indicates functional activity, or a "cold" nodule, which indicates no functional activity. Hot nodules are rarely malignant; cold nodules may be malignant. Laboratory tests are minimally helpful in establishing a diagnosis of thyroid cancer, with the exception of serum calcitonin level measurement if medullary thyroid cancer is suspected. A family history of thyroid cancer should raise the suspicion of multiple endocrine neoplasia type I and thus a serum calcitonin level should be measured. An FNA biopsy is a valuable aid in establishing a diagnosis and thus in determining the appropriate management of a thyroid nodule. The diagnostic accuracy of aspiration cytologic testing is 71% to 92% and depends on the experience of the operator and the pathologist. In aspiration cytologic testing of the thyroid, the patient is placed in the supine position and a pillow is placed under the shoulders to extend the neck; this increases exposure of the thyroid gland. The physician should stand at the patient's side ipsilateral or contralateral to the lesion. The entire thyroid is palpated to determine the size and location of any abnormalities. The skin is cleansed with alcohol. Some clinicians recommend that the skin and soft tissues over the intended aspiration site be infiltrated with 1% or 2% lidocaine to allow adequate sampling. A gentle massage of the soft tissues of the neck allows for dispersal of the injected fluid and avoids obscuring the thyroid nodule. However, some authorities avoid using the local anesthetic because of the possibility that it may obscure the outlines of the lesion and make aspiration more difficult. A 25-gauge 1-inch disposable needle is attached to a 10-mL syringe with a pistol handle and used initially (Fig. 2-3). One milliliter of air is drawn into the syringe before aspiration to facilitate expelling the specimen. The lesion is fixed between the thumb and index finger or the index and middle fingers of a sterile

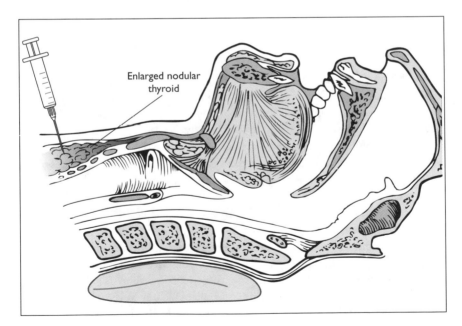

Enlarged nodular thyroid

Figure 2-3 Aspiration of the thyroid gland.

gloved hand, and the needle is placed in the center of a small nodule (1 to 2 cm) or in the periphery of a large nodule (2 to 4 cm). When the needle is believed to be within the nodule, suction is applied on the plunger of the syringe. While maintaining suction, the needle is quickly moved back and forth with short strokes in the same tract. The procedure is stopped when material appears in the needle hub or after 6 to 10 strokes. The vacuum is released before the needle is withdrawn. Pressure is applied to the neck to minimize hematoma formation.

With the needle bevel pointing down, one or two drops of the aspirated material is expressed onto a clean slide. To make a smear, a new clean slide is gently placed on top of the slide that holds the material droplets and the two slides are gently pulled apart in a horizontal plane. The slides are allowed to air-dry. The remainder of the material is recovered by rinsing the syringe with Cytolyte® solution.

The old needle is discarded. A new needle is placed onto the 10-mL syringe, and the process is repeated. Three to six aspirations should be performed. Overall, FNA of the thyroid gland is extremely safe, and the risk of tumor seeding the tract is 1 in 20,000.

The trachea may be entered during the FNA procedure, which may provoke a cough or even blood-tinged sputum; however, tracheal puncture does not lead to long-term sequelae.

Similarly, FNA is a useful method in the work-up of a dominant mass within the breast. If a dominant mass is found that has a cystic quality to it, it is perfectly permissible to attempt FNA, keeping in mind that one should outline to the patient an alternate plan if the aspiration does not yield fluid. The alternate should be implemented promptly if an attempt at aspiration is unsuccessful. The skin is prepped with alcohol or povidone-iodine (Betadine®). The skin is infiltrated with 1% or 2% lidocaine, and the lump is positioned between two fingers of a sterile gloved hand. A 21- to 23-gauge 1.5-inch disposable needle attached to a 5- or 10-mL syringe is inserted into the center of the mass, and the syringe is aspirated. If clear fluid is recovered, it is discarded; if bloody fluid is aspirated, it should be placed in Cytolyte® solution and sent to the pathology laboratory. If no fluid is aspirated, the syringe should be rinsed with Cytolyte® and the contents sent to the cytology laboratory. The false-negative rate of FNAs is 9.6%.

Fine-needle aspiration is the preferred approach in the work-up of a "coin" lesion within the lung. The solitary pulmonary nodule, or "coin" lesion, is found on a routine chest radiograph in an otherwise asymptomatic individual. Once a coin lesion is discovered, the next diagnostic step is computed tomography (CT) of the chest to confirm the presence of a single nodule (as opposed to multiple nodules) and to confirm the presence of calcifications, which if present imply old granulomatous disease. If a solitary nodule is not calcified, a CT-guided FNA is the next step. The FNA yields an answer 92% of the time, with a false-negative rate of 34%.

Fine-needle aspiration is a useful approach in the work-up of suspected prostate cancer. If a nodule is palpable within the prostate, urologic referral and an ultrasonography-guided transrectal FNA of the nodule and prostate is a useful approach. However, in many men, the most important indicator of any prostate disease is an elevated screening serum prostate-specific antigen (PSA [also see Chapter 11, p 177]). The prostate may feel diffusely firm or normal on digital examination. In such an instance, urologic referral and ultrasonography-guided FNA yields a diagnosis of prostate cancer with 90% accuracy.

Excisional Biopsies

Although FNAs are clearly useful and relatively noninvasive, there are instances when an excisional biopsy should be performed. As discussed earlier in this chapter, the occurrence of lymphadenopathy (lymph nodes >1 cm except in the inguinal region) indicates a pathologic process. *Persistent lymphadenopathy for more than 6 weeks* without a known underlying cause or supraclavicular lymphadenopathy of any size or duration requires excisional biopsy. The justification for excisional biopsy is that, with lymphomas, the architecture of the lymphoma (follicular or diffuse) is as important as the individual cellular proliferation (e.g., small lymphocytic, small-cleaved cell, large cell). The manner in which the lymph node is handled by the surgeon is important. I advise surgeons to take the fresh node to the pathology laboratory rather than place the node in fixative (formalin). The pathologist usually cuts the node in half, reserving half and freezing it so that it is available for future testing and processing the other half in the usual manner.

The other instance in which excisional biopsy is indicated is in the clinical setting of a breast mass when an FNA has not yielded a diagnosis. Although FNA cytologic testing clearly has a role in the evaluation of a dominant breast mass, its failure to obtain a diagnosis is an indication for a timely and expedient excisional biopsy. Because women of all ages fear breast cancer, waiting for a test to be scheduled or for test results is extremely anxiety provoking for them. Therefore, scheduling tests promptly and relating test results in a timely way can only lessen the anxiety. In premenopausal women with a breast mass in whom an FNA does not yield a diagnosis, ultrasonography and referral to a general surgeon for excisional biopsy is the proper recourse. In postmenopausal women, mammography and surgical referral is the appropriate approach.

Endoscopic Biopsy

Endoscopic examination clearly plays a role in the evaluation of hilar masses, gastrointestinal bleeding, and hematuria. If a hilar mass is disclosed on chest radiography, bronchoscopy and biopsy, either endobronchial or transbronchial, is the preferred approach. Bronchoscopy and biopsy not only yield information on the histologic features of the disease but also on its proximity to the carina.

Esophagoscopy, gastroscopy, duodenoscopy, and/or colonoscopy are all useful procedures in defining the cause of upper or lower gastrointestinal bleeding. In the work-up of bright red rectal bleeding (BRRB) or Hematest-positive stool, colonoscopy is the procedure of choice. Colonoscopy defines the cause of the BRRB in 98% of cases. If a diagnosis of colonic cancer is made, surgical referral is appropriate, even in the setting of known metastasis, to avoid colonic obstruction. Similarly, in the work-up of occult gastrointestinal bleeding (Hematest-positive stool) colonoscopy and upper endoscopy are necessary to determine the cause. Case 2-1 illustrates the value of endoscopy.

Case 2-1

Mrs. Y.S. is an 86-year-old woman with a long-standing history of polycythemia rubra vera (PRV) treated with periodic phlebotomy. She had excellent control of PRV for many years. In 1997, she was found to have thrombocytosis, 1,100,000 platelets/μL. Her hemoglobin level was 12.3 g/dL; the mean cellular volume (MCV) was 62, and the reticulocyte count was 0.5%. Her previous hemoglobin level was 13.9 g/dL, with an MCV of 75 and platelets of 495,000 cells/μL The physical examination, including rectal examination, was unremarkable, and the spleen was not palpable. The results of a stool test for occult blood at the time of the physical examination were negative. Her serum ferritin level was measured and she was asked to go on a meat-free diet for 3 days, obtain stool for occult blood testing, and return in 1 week. The clinical suspicion was that she had become increasingly iron deficient owing to occult gastrointestinal (GI) bleeding and that the GI bleeding and worsening iron deficiency led to the thrombocytosis. She returned in 1 week. The serum ferritin was 5 mg/dL, and two of the three stool specimens were Hematest-positive. She was referred to a gastroenterologist who performed a colonoscopy and found a cecal carcinoma. She subsequently underwent a right hemicolectomy and was found to have colonic carcinoma stage B1.

Discussion
Despite her PRV, this woman's case history illustrates several different points that can be generalized as follows:

1. Thrombocytosis and a change in hemoglobin must be explained. Although her hemoglobin level at presentation was "normal," the decrease in the hemoglobin level by 1 g was significant. A decrease in the hemoglobin level coupled with thrombocytosis and a decrease in the MCV must be considered blood loss until proven otherwise. Even if the stools had been Hematest-negative, a GI work-up would have been necessary before one would consider performing a repeat bone marrow examination.

2. After GI blood loss was documented, a colonoscopy yielded a diagnosis. Had the colonoscopy been nondiagnostic, an esophagogastroduodenoscopy would have been performed.

The presence of hematuria should prompt an abdominal-pelvic CT to rule out a kidney neoplasm. After this has been done, the patient should be referred to a urologist and cystoscopy should be carried out. If detected early, bladder cancer is highly curable.

Histologic Analysis

An experienced pathologist examining a hematoxylin and eosin (H&E) stained tissue specimen under light microscopy and aided with a clinical history (communication with the primary care physician is essential; pathologists should not be expected to render a diagnosis in a vacuum) should in most cases provide a pathologic diagnosis. Additional histologic analysis such as nuclear grade, degree of differentiation, Gleason score, and so on may provide useful prognostic information as well as information that will guide decisions regarding therapy. Histologic grading should be done routinely for the malignancies shown in Table 2-2.

The histologic and nuclear grading systems use scores of I to IV, with grade I representing the best degree of differentiation or nuclear grade and with grade IV representing the worst. The Gleason score is routinely used in patients with prostate cancer. The Gleason score is a five-point scheme, with a score of 1 representing well-differentiated prostate cancer and with 5 representing undifferentiated prostate cancer. The pathologist examines the prostate specimen and assigns a score to the most well-differentiated portion and to the least differentiated portion. The two most prevalent scores are added together and yield an overall score of 2 to 10. Fundamentally, scores of 2 and 3 represent well-differentiated prostate cancer; 4 to 6, moderately differentiated cancer; 7 to 9, poorly differentiated cancer; and 10, undifferentiated cancer.

Similarly, in breast cancer, the degree of nuclear grade correlates with the estrogen and progesterone receptor content and correlates with disease-free and overall survival. Although nuclear grade is not an independent prognostic factor, it does provide information as to the biology of a given breast cancer. Breast cancers with a nuclear grade I are low-grade malignancies; breast cancers with a nuclear grade IV are biologically aggressive. Assessment of nuclear grade plays an important role in adjuvant therapy decisions.

Table 2-2 Histologic Grading That Should Be Done Routinely in the Histologic Assessment of Malignancy

Malignancy	Grading System
Head and neck	Degree of differentiation
Lung, adenocarcinoma	Degree of differentiation
Breast	Nuclear grade
Prostate	Gleason score
Sarcomas	Degree of differentiation

An additional pathologic determinant in breast cancer that is an independent prognostic factor is the presence or absence of vascular invasion. The presence of vascular invasion predicts for a poorer disease-free and overall survival. In order to access for vascular invasion, immunohistochemical stains directed against factor VIII, which is synthesized in endothelial cells, need to be performed to outline blood vessels accurately. The number of invaded blood vessels are counted. Women with greater than 100 invaded blood vessels tend to have a poorer overall prognosis.

In patients with soft tissue sarcomas, the degree of differentiation influences decisions regarding the need for adjuvant chemotherapy. Low-grade (grade I or II) liposarcomas have low metastatic potential, and systemic adjuvant chemotherapy is not needed. Adjuvant chemotherapy is reserved for higher-grade liposarcomas (grades III or IV).

Cancer of Unknown Primary Origin

In most instances, the histologic diagnosis of malignancy and its site of origin are straightforward. At other times, however, the site of origin is obscure even though the diagnosis of malignancy is straightforward. In such cases, a diagnosis of cancer of unknown primary origin (CUP) is made. Communication between the attending physician and the pathologist is very important. Although the initial impulse is to perform "head to toe scans" and endoscopic procedures in search of the primary origin, one must bear in mind that a more thoughtful approach coupled with immunohistochemical stains, molecular marker studies, and cytogenetic studies is more likely to yield answers.

The definition of CUP is metastatic disease in the absence of a discernible primary site after a complete medical history, careful physical examination, chest radiography, complete blood count, multichannel serum chemistries, stool occult blood testing, urinalysis, and computed tomography of the abdomen and pelvis have been done. The primary site may be "too small" or slow growing to declare itself, or the primary site may have undergone spontaneous regression owing to immunologic mechanisms. Histologically, patients with CUP are divided into four major categories (Table 2-3): (1) those with adenocarcinomas (the most common category of CUP); (2) those with poorly differentiated carcinomas (the second most common category of CUP); (3) squamous cell carcinomas that present with metastases to cervical lymph nodes in the absence of a discernible primary site; and (4) undifferentiated malignant neoplasms. With the aid of additional immunohistochemical tests, undifferentiated malignant neoplasms are frequently latter classified as poorly differentiated carcinomas, malignant lymphomas, malignant melanoma, or sarcomas.

CUP accounts for approximately 3% of all cancer diagnoses in the United States and presents a difficult challenge to primary care physicians.

Table 2-3 Histologic Subsets of Cancer of Unknown Primary Origin*

Adenocarcinoma, well to moderately differentiated
Poorly differentiated carcinomas and adenocarcinomas
Squamous cell carcinoma
Undifferentiated malignant neoplasms of an undiscernible primary[†]

*In descending order of frequency.
[†]Undifferentiated malignant neoplasms are frequently later classified as poorly differentiated carcinomas, malignant lymphomas, malignant melanoma, or sarcomas with the aid of additional immunohistochemical tests.

Although the natural history of patients with CUP is aggressive and the overall prognosis is poor (median survival of 5 to 10 months), there are some notable exceptions and therefore it is important to formulate a careful and thoughtful diagnostic plan. In the past, the diagnostic approach to patients with CUP was to perform an all-encompassing radiologic work-up without regard to the clinical symptoms. Patients with CUP underwent needless and low-yield radiography studies in an attempt to uncover the primary tumor. Clearly, this approach was wrong then and is wrong now. Currently, the diagnostic approach to patients with CUP is based on the presenting symptoms, physical findings, and the pathologic features of the CUP. Emphasis is placed on the pathologic findings. Immunohistochemical stains, cytogenetic studies, and, occasionally, serum marker studies are used to find the primary site. It is recognized that, despite a reasonable work-up, in most patients with CUP the primary site is never identified (Fig. 2-4). Routine immunohistochemical stains performed on biopsy material include common leukocyte antigen (leukemia/lymphoma), carcinoembryonic antigen (CEA, carcinomas), cytokeratin (carcinomas), and vimentin (sarcoma, melanoma, lymphoma).

Based on the results of the initial routine immunohistochemical stains, the pathologist may wish to do additional immunohistochemical stains or to perform molecular studies to identify definitively the primary site. For example, in a patient with an undifferentiated malignancy involving a lymph node that stains initially for the common leukocyte antigen, additional immunohistochemical stains with monoclonal antibodies to CD19 and CD20 (both B-lymphocyte antigens), CD3, CD4, CD8 (all T-lymphocyte antigens) should be done to conclusively prove the presence of a malignant lymphoma and to determine whether it is a T-cell or B-cell lymphoma. If the undifferentiated malignancy failed to stain with these monoclonal antibodies, the pathologist could perform molecular studies looking for a rearranged T-cell receptor gene or a rearranged immunoglobulin light-chain gene in an attempt to prove conclusively the presence of a lymphoma. A variety of clinical situations and the steps involved in the diagnostic work-up are shown in Table 2-4. Case 2-2 illustrates the approach to women with cancer in axillary lymph nodes.

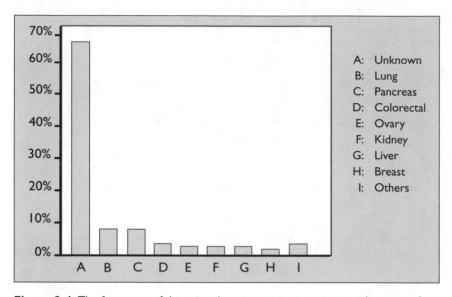

Figure 2-4 The frequency of detecting the primary site in patients with cancer of unknown primary origin. As shown by the bar graph, in most patients, the primary site remains unknown.

Table 2-4 What to Consider in the Diagnostic Work-up of Selected Patients with Cancer of Unknown Primary Origin

Clinical Situation	Histology	Need to Rule Out	Next Diagnostic Steps
Young men or women with mediastinal masses	Undifferentiated cancer	Extragonadal germ cell cancer	Serum AFP, β-HCG, stains for AFP and cytokeratin
Young men or women with pelvic masses	Undifferentiated cancer	Neuroblastoma	Urine HVA and VMA, cytogenetics
Women with cancer in axillary lymph nodes	Adenocarcinoma	Breast cancer	ER/PR, CA 27.29
Women with ascites	Adenocarcinoma	Ovarian cancer	ER/PR, CA-125
Men with bone or lung metastasis	Adenocarcinoma	Prostate cancer	Serum PSA, stain for PSA
Men or women with lung nodules, hilar or mediastinal masses	Adenocarcinoma	Lung cancer	Stain for cytokeratin
Men or women with single or multiple liver masses	Adenocarcinoma	Hepatoma	Serum AFP, CEA
Men or (rarely) women with enlarged cervical lymph nodes	Squamous cell cancer	Head and neck cancer	Stain for cytokeratin

AFP = α-fetoprotein; HCG = human chorionic gonadotropin; HVA = homovanillic acid; VMA = vanillylmandelic acid; ER = estrogen receptor; PR = progesterone receptor; PSA = prostate-specific antigen; CEA = carcinoembryonic antigen.

Case 2.2

A 47-year-old single woman presents to her physician with a right axillary mass. The physical findings reveal an enlarged (2 × 3 cm), firm, moveable lymph node within the right axilla. No other lymph nodes are palpable, and a careful examination of both breasts fails to reveal any dominant lumps. The remainder of the physical examation is unremarkable. The patient is premenopausal, gravida 0, para 0, and has no history of breast cancer. Bilateral mammography fails to reveal any abnormalities. Excisional biopsy of the right axillary node reveals a metastatic, poorly differentiated adenocarcinoma consistent with a breast primary site. The nodal metastasis does not express estrogen or progesterone receptors. Chest radiography reveals no abnormalities, and the results of multichannel chemistries are normal.

The patient undergoes a modified right radical mastectomy. The pathologic features of the breast specimen do not reveal any breast cancer. The patient receives treatment with four cycles of cyclophosphamide and doxorubicin. She is currently in her seventh year of follow-up and remains disease free.

Cytogenetics and Molecular Studies

As discussed in Chapter 1 (in the section "Cancer Genetics"), specific chromosomal abnormalities (e.g., translocations, deletions, inversions) are associated with specific malignancies (see Table 1-5, p 16). Chromosomal abnormalities do play an increasingly important role in the diagnosis of malignancy. For example, the microgranular variant of acute promyelocytic leukemia (APL) cannot be distinguished histologically from other forms of acute myeloid leukemia; however, the microgranular form of APL can be diagnosed with the use of chromosomal analysis, which always shows the 15/17 translocation. The differential diagnosis of "small blue tumors of bone" includes Ewing sarcoma, neuroblastoma, Wilm tumor, and lymphoma. The diagnosis of each of these is readily aided by cytogenetic analysis. As shown in Table 1-5, the cytogenetic abnormalities differ for these individual malignancies, and chromosomal analysis would aid in the differential diagnosis.

Molecular studies already play a role in the complete pathologic evaluation of a malignancy. In the future, molecular studies will play an increasingly important role not only in defining the biologic aggressiveness or indolence of a given malignancy but also in establishing a diagnosis or assessing the adequacy of the margins of resection. It is now routine to measure estrogen receptor (ER) and progesterone receptor (PR) content in breast cancer. These nuclear receptors play an important role in the proliferation and the differentiation of normal breast ductal cells. When ER and PR are expressed in significantly elevated levels in women with breast cancer, these patients have an overall better prognosis than their ER- and PR-negative counterparts. The usefulness of ER and PR measurement is not confined solely to the management of breast cancer. Estrogen and progesterone receptors are expressed by uterine endometrial cells, ovarian stromal cells and oocytes, the cellular lining of the fallopian tube, and occasionally by malignant melanoma and colon cancer. As shown in Table 2-5, the measurement of ER and PR can play a diagnostic role in women with CUP who present with either an enlarged unilateral axillary lymph node or malignant ascites with or without a pelvic mass. In the latter setting, it may be difficult to differentiate a cancer of the sigmoid colon with extension into the pelvis from an ovarian cancer with extension into the sigmoid colon. The presence of ER or PR would make a diagnosis of ovarian cancer more likely and that of colon cancer far less likely. As the treatment and prognosis of ovarian cancer are vastly different than those of colon cancer, arriving at the most accurate diagnosis is critical. The androgen receptor is typically expressed in prostate cancer; however, to date there is no role for its routine assay. Steroid receptors are expressed normally in lymphocytes and in neoplastic lymphocytes, lymphoblastic leukemia, and lymphomas. The assay for steroid receptors in leukemias and lymphomas has no clinical import. It does not help with the diagnosis or prognosis.

Although assays for ER and PR are one type of molecular analysis, assays for overexpressed or mutant oncogenes are another. In the future, molecular studies will supplement histologic examination or, in some instances, supersede conventional histologic examination (Table 2-6). Currently, most of the pathology laboratories in the United States are testing for *Her-2/neu* overexpression in breast cancer (see Chapter 1, the section "Oncogenes," pp 9–15). The overexpression of *Her-2/neu* confers a poor prognosis in both breast and ovarian cancer. Patients with adenocarcinoma of the lung with a mutant K-*ras* oncogene have a poorer prognosis than do patients with adenocarcinoma of the lung with the "wild-type" K-*ras*. The overexpression of *bcl-2* confers a more favorable prognosis in patients with malignant lymphomas and breast cancer. Recent studies in head and neck cancer have shown that the adjacent "normal epithelium" surrounding a resected head and neck cancer may harbor a mutant p53 gene, which typically represents a premalignant finding. Assaying for mutant p53 may give head and neck surgeons a better guide as to the adequacy of the resected margins. As more light is shed on the molecular

Table 2-5 Carcinomas that Commonly Express Estrogen and Progesterone Receptors

Breast cancer
Ovarian cancer
Endometrial cancer
Adenocarcinoma of the fallopian tube

Table 2-6 Additional Studies Including Molecular Analysis to Accompany Routine Histologic Analysis

Malignancy	Additional Studies
Head and neck cancer	Mutant p53 at surgical margins
Breast cancer	ER/PR, *Her-2/neu* overexpression, presence of vascular invasion
Adenocarcinoma of the lung	K-*ras* mutation
Ovarian cancer	*Her-2/neu* overexpression
Prostate cancer	Gleason score
Lymphoma	B-cell/T-cell markers, *bcl*-2 overexpression
Leukemias	Cytogenetics (chromosomal analysis)
Bladder and gastric cancer, sarcomas	Degree of differentiation

ER = estrogen receptor; PR = progesterone receptor.

biology of cancer, molecular testing will become part of the routine pathologic work-up in the future.

Serum Markers

The hope continues that someday a blood test will become available for screening patients for a clinically occult malignancy or, alternatively, for the testing and follow up of patients with malignancies. To date, this hope has become a reality only in prostate cancer. Prostate-specific antigen is the only serum marker that is used in the screening for prostate cancer and in the staging, treatment evaluation, and follow-up of men with prostate cancer. Other serum markers such as carcinoembryonic antigen (CEA), CA-125, CA 27.29, α-fetoprotein, and the β-subunit of human chorionic gonadotropin (β-HCG) are not to be used in the screening for malignancy because in general they are insensitive and have low specificity.

Prostate-specific antigen is a serine protease produced by benign and malignant prostate epithelium. It is measured by radioimmunoassay, and although PSA *is prostate specific it is not cancer specific.* Prostatitis, benign prostatic hypertrophy, and prostate manipulation are all capable of causing an elevation of PSA. The serum half-life of PSA is approximately 3 days. Currently, PSA is the only serum marker that received FDA approval for the screening and early detection of prostate cancer. It is important to recognize that as men age, an increase in PSA occurs owing to benign prostatic hypertrophy; therefore, many experts prefer to use age-adjusted PSA (Table 2-7).

As shown in Table 2-7, in men older than 70 years an abnormal PSA is one that exceeds 6.5 ng/mL. Using age-adjusted PSA may decrease the number of

Table 2-7 "Age Adjusted" Prostate-Specific Antigen (PSA)

Age Range (yr)	Serum PSA (ng/mL)
40–49	0–2.5
50–59	0–3.5
60–69	0–4.5
70–79	0–6.5

Adapted from Oesterling JE, Jacobsen GJ, Chute CG. Prostate-specific antigen: improving its ability to diagnose early prostate cancer [Editorial]. JAMA. 1992;267:2236-8.

Table 2-8 Predictive Values of Digital Rectal Examination (DRE) and Prostate-Specific Antigen (PSA)

DRE	PSA (ng/mL)	Positive Predictive Value
Any finding	4.1–4.9	26%
Any finding	>10	53%
Abnormal	<4	10%
Abnormal	>4	48.5%
Normal	4.1–4.9	21.7%
Normal	>10	42.2%

Adapted from Ohori M, Scardino PT. Early detection of prostate cancer: the nature of cancers detected with current diagnostic tests. Semin Oncol. 1994;21:522-6.

diagnostic work-ups that are otherwise prompted by screening. Screening for prostate cancer involves both a digital rectal examination (DRE) and measurement of serum PSA. Screening should be done yearly in men older than 50 years, and in those considered to be at high risk for the disease (African-American men and men with a family history of prostate cancer), annual screening should begin at age 40 years. The predictive values of an abnormal PSA level and of abnormal DRE results are shown in Table 2-8.

As shown in this table, when the results of the DRE are normal and the PSA level is elevated (4.1–4.9 ng/mL), the probability of prostate cancer is 21.7%. If the PSA level is more than 10 ng/mL, the probability is 42.2%. In contrast, when the results of the DRE are abnormal (a nodule and/or firm area are found) and the PSA level is less than 4 ng/mL, the probability of prostate cancer is only 10%. Men with a serum PSA level of more than 10 ng/mL and with normal findings on DRE have a 42% probability of prostate cancer.

A clear-cut relation exists between the PSA level and cancer stage. As shown in Tables 2-9 and 2-10, the PSA level does correlate with the extent of disease. Men with a serum PSA level that exceeds 40 ng/mL likely have extracapsular extension (stage C) or metastatic prostate cancer (stage D). Similarly, although a

Table 2-9 Serum Prostate-Specific Antigen (PSA) Values and Their Relation to the Stage of Prostate Cancer

Stage	Serum PSA (ng/mL)
A I and A2 (inapparent tumor, T I)	4–8
B (confined to prostate, T2)	12–40
C (extracapsular extension, T3 or T4)	40–60
D I or D2 (nodal or visceral involvement)	40–200+

Table 2-10 Relation Between Serum Prostate-Specific Antigen (PSA) and Pathologic Stage in Men with "Localized" Prostate Cancer

Serum PSA (ng/mL)	No. of Patients	Prostate-Confined	Capsular Spread	Seminal Vesicles Involved	Seminal Vesicle or Nodal Involvement
0–4	421	325 (77%)	81 (9%)	8 (2%)	8 (2%)
4–10	533	324 (61%)	153 (29%)	19 (3%)	37 (7%)
10–20	311	139 (45%)	94 (30%)	38 (12%)	40 (13%)
>20	251	67 (27%)	63 (25%)	52 (20%)	78 (28%)

Republished from Trump DL, Shipley WU, Dilloglugil O, Scardino P. Neoplasms of the prostate. In: Holland JF, Frei E, Bast RO Jr, et al., eds. Cancer Medicine. 4th ed. Baltimore: Williams and Wilkins; 1997:2134.

serum PSA level of more than 20 ng/mL is associated with a lesser probability of extracapsular spread or nodal involvement, only 27% of patients have disease confined to the prostate. Serum PSA helps in defining the extent of disease.

After appropriate treatment has been determined (see Chapter 11), measurement of the PSA is valuable in evaluating the efficacy of therapy and in follow-up. If hormonal therapy is used and the patient responds to this treatment, the PSA should promptly decrease within 60 days. Persistent elevation of the PSA or a decrease that is less than 75% of the pretreatment value implies resistance to therapy. Similarly, after surgery or after the completion of radiotherapy (with or without radioactive seed implants), the PSA should decrease to normal values within 60 days. Measurement of the PSA level is also the most sensitive means of detecting recurrent prostate cancer, even more so than a periodic physical examination. If the serum PSA level is found to be elevated, it should be measured again within 3 to 4 weeks. A persistently elevated PSA level indicates recurrent disease, and the search for the site of recurrence should be begun (see Chapter 11, p 177).

Carcinoembryonic antigen is a protein-polysaccharide complex found in colonic cancers and in the normal fetal gut, pancreas, and liver. Carcinoembryonic antigen can be oversynthesized by colonic cancer, breast cancer, lung cancer, gastric cancer, endometrial cancer, and cervical cancer. Accordingly, the specificity of CEA is low and elevated levels (>3.5 ng/mL and <10 ng/mL) can occur in heavy cigarette smokers, in persons with cirrhosis, and in persons with ulcerative colitis. A CEA of more than 10 ng/mL is usually associated with a malignant process. Periodic monitoring of CEA is useful in detecting recurrences of colonic cancer. Additionally, a serum CEA level should be obtained as a baseline in women with breast cancer and bone metastases, and, if elevated, CEA is useful in monitoring the efficacy of therapy (for both hormonal therapy and chemotherapy).

CA 27.29 is a high–molecular weight glycoprotein (mucins) expressed in the membrane of breast cancer cells. When the standard cutoff of less than 35 U/µL is used, an elevated serum CA 27.29 level can be found in women with benign breast disease (8%) and hepatitis (30%), in addition to those with breast cancer. An elevated serum CA 27.29 has low sensitivity (31%) for malignant breast disease but relatively high specificity (86%) and diagnostic accuracy (81%). It is a very good marker for detecting recurrent disease in women with breast cancer. It is helpful in evaluating the response to therapy in women with metastatic breast cancer who have nonmeasurable disease such as predominantly bone metastases. A decrease of more than 50% from baseline value indicates a response to therapy; an increase of more than 25% indicates disease progression.

CA-125 is a 200-kD glycoprotein found as a surface glycoprotein in ovarian cancer. When a cutoff of 35 U/µL is used, an elevated CA-125 level is found in 1% of normal women, 6% of women with benign ovarian tumors or endometriosis, 12% of women with breast cancer, 21% of women with colorectal cancer, 32% of women with lung cancer, 59% of women with pancreatic cancer, and 86% of women with ovarian cancer. CA-125 is a valuable tool in determining the response to chemotherapy and in follow-up of women with ovarian cancer. CA-125 is not useful in screening women for ovarian cancer because of its low specificity. However, CA-125 coupled with endovaginal ultrasonography should be used for ovarian cancer screening in women who are genetically predisposed, such as those who are carriers of *BRCA1*.

α-Fetoprotein (AFP) is a normal protein product of fetal liver cells. Elevated levels may be found in the serum of patients with primary hepatoma, testis cancer (embryonal cell carcinoma, malignant teratomas, and yolk-sac tumors), and germ cell tumors of the ovary. AFP has a half-life of 7 days. Baseline levels should be obtained in men with testis cancer and in women with germ cell tumors. An elevated level that does not return to normal within 14 days of surgical resection indicates more extensive disease. In patients with germ cell tumors, AFP is useful in monitoring the response to chemotherapy and in determining the persistence of disease after retroperitoneal node dissection. An elevated AFP level after retroperitoneal node dissection indicates serologic stage III disease. After the completion of therapy, AFP is useful in monitoring for the presence of recurrent disease.

β-HCG is measured by radioimmunoassay and has a half-life of 24 hours. β-HCG has a role in the management of women with gestational trophoblastic neoplasms (GTN). (Gestational trophoblastic neoplasms is a disease spectrum that includes hydatidiform moles, nonmetastatic GTN, and metastatic GTN [choriocarcinoma]) The β-subunit is specific for HCG. The β-subunit cross-reacts with human luteinizing hormone, follicle-stimulating hormone, and thyroid-stimulating hormone. β-HCG is elevated in men with testis cancer, embryonal cell cancer, yolk-sac tumors, choriocarcinoma, and germ cell tumors of the ovary.

Other markers, such as CA 19-9, a purported marker for pancreatic cancer, offer little in the management of patients with pancreatic cancer and cannot be recommended for clinical use at this time.

Chapter 3

Cancer Staging and Diagnostics

C ancer therapy cannot be initiated until an unequivocal diagnosis of malignancy has been made. A variety of classification systems are used in the staging of cancer. These classification systems stage cancer based on the anatomic extent of disease. Staging allows physicians to make appropriate treatment decisions, furnishes prognostic information, and provides a common language that may be used by clinical investigators.

The staging classification proposed by the American Joint Committee on Cancer (AJCC) is the most widely used in the United States and overlaps with a system proposed by the International Union Against Cancer. The anatomic extent of disease is based on tumor size (T), nodal status (N), and the presence or absence of distant metastases (M). Examples of the AJCC staging classifications of some of the more common epithelial malignancies are shown in Tables 3-1 through 3-6. As these tables show, some staging classifications are based on clinical findings (lung, breast, and lymphoma, Tables 3-1 and 3-6), some are strictly based on pathologic findings (colorectal and gastric, Tables 3-1 and 3-5), and some others are based on a combination of both (bladder, prostate, esophageal, pancreas, testis, kidney, ovary, and endometrium, Tables 3-1 through 3-6).

The staging of head and neck cancer is grounded solely on clinical findings. Squamous cell carcinoma of the lip and oral cavity begins as a mucosal lesion that slowly invades the tissues of the oral cavity. Involvement of the regional lymph nodes or distant metastases occurs late and correlates with the size of the primary tumor. A carcinoma in situ is considered stage 0.

Table 3-1 Staging of Lung, Breast,

	Lung Cancer	Breast Cancer
Primary Tumor		
Tis	Carcinoma in situ	Ductal carcinoma in situ
T1	Tumor <3 cm surrounded by lung or visceral pleura	Tumor <2 cm (T1a <5 mm, T1b = 5–9 mm, T1c >10 mm)
T2	Tumor >3 cm or invasion of visceral pleura, or obstructive pneumonitis	Tumor >2 cm <5 cm
T3	Tumor of any size with invasion of chest wall, diaphragm, esophagus, or with 2 cm of carina	Tumor >5 cm
T4	Tumor with invasion of mediastinal structures or malignant pleural effusion	Tumor of any size with extension to chest wall
T5	N/A	N/A
Nodal Involvement		
N0	No regional nodal metastases	No palpable ipsilateral axillary nodes
N1	Metastasis to ipsilateral peribronchial or hilar nodes	Movable ipsilateral axillary lymph nodes N1a: no clinical metastases N1b: clinical metastases
N2	Metastases to ipsilateral mediastinal nodes	Fixed and matted axillary nodes
N3	Contralateral mediastinal nodes	Supraclavicular or infraclavicular nodes
Metastases		
M0	No distant metastases	No distant metastases
M1	Distant metastases	Distant metastases
Staging		
Stage 0	Tis, N0, M0	Tis, N0, M0
Stage I	T1 or T2, N0, M0	T1, N0, N1a, M0
Stage II	T1 or T2, N1, M0	T0 or T1, N1b, M0 T2, N1a, N1b, M0
Stage IIIa	T3, N0, N1, M0	T3, N0, N1 or N2, M0
Stage IIIb	T1–3, N2, M0	Inflammatory carcinoma
Stage IV	Any T, any N, M1	T4 or N3 or M1

N/A = not applicable; PSA = prostate-specific antigen.

Colon, and Prostate Cancers

	Colon Cancer	Prostate Cancer
	Carcinoma in situ	N/A
	Tumor confined to mucosa or sub-mucosa	Clinically occult (T1a <5% of chips, T1b >5% of chips, T1c = positive needle biopsy with elevated PSA)
	Invasion of muscularis up to serosa	Confined to prostate (T2a <half lobe, T2b >half lobe, T2c = both lobes)
	Invasion through serosa or adjacent organs	Extracapsular invasion
	Fistula formation	Fixed or invasion of adjacent structures
	Extension beyond adjacent organs	N/A
	No nodal metastases	No nodal metastases
	Any nodal involvement	Single node <2 cm
	N/A	Single node >2 cm <5 cm
	N/A	Single node >5 cm
	No distant metastases	No distant metastases
	Distant metastases	Distant metastases

Staging

	Colon Cancer	Prostate Cancer
Stage 0	Tis, N0, M0	N/A
Stage A	T1, N0, M0	T1, N0, M0
Stage B		T2, N0, M0
Stage B1	T2, N0, M0	
Stage B2	T3–5, N0, M0	
Stage C		T3, N0, M0
Stage C1	T1 or T2, N1, M0	
Stage C2	T3 or T4, N1, M0	
Stage D	Any T, any N, M1	
Stage D1		Any T, N1–3, M0
Stage D2		Any T, any N, M1

Table 3-2 Staging of Bladder, Kidney, and Testis Cancer

	Bladder	Testis	Kidney
Stage 0a	Noninvasive papillary cancer	—	—
Stage 0is	Carcinoma in situ (flat tumor)	—	—
Stage I	Involvement of subepithelial connective tissue	Tumor confined to testis	Tumor confined to kidney; no perinephric involvement
Stage II	Muscle invasion, superficial or deep	Nodal involvement A. Lymph nodes <2 cm B. Lymph nodes >2 cm <5 cm C. Lymph nodes >5 cm	Tumor involving perinephric fat but confined to Gerota fascia; no invasion of renal vein or renal lymph nodes
Stage III	Invasion of perivascular fat, prostate, uterus, or vagina	Supradiaphragmatic involvement	Invasion of renal veins or perirenal lymph nodes
Stage IV	Involvement of pelvis, abdominal wall, lymph nodes, or distant metastases	Visceral metastases	Distant metastases

Table 3-3 Staging of Endometrial and Ovarian Cancer

Stage	Endometrial Cancer	Ovarian Cancer
IA	Confined to the endometrium	Confined to one ovary
IB	Involvement of less than one half of the myometrium	Confined to both ovaries
IC	Involvement of more than one half of the myometrium	Extracapsular extension or positive cytologic findings
IIA	Extension to the endocervix	Involvement of the uterus or fallopian tubes
IIB	Extension into cervical stroma	Involvement of other parametrial tissues
IIC		As above with positive cytologic findings
IIIA	Extension into serosa and/or positive cytologic findings	Involvement of the true pelvis with abdominal metastases
IIIB	Extension into vagina	Abdominal metastases <2 cm
IIIC	Lymph nodal involvement, pelvic or para-aortic	Abdominal metastases >2 cm
IV		Visceral metastases
IVA	Bladder or bowel invasion	
IVB	Visceral metastases	

Stage 1 is assigned to cancer in which patients have tumors that are less than 2 cm in size (T1) and have no palpable lymph nodes (N0) and no distant metastasis (M0). Cancer in which tumors are greater than 2 cm in size but less than 4 cm (T2) and in which there are no palpable lymph nodes (N0) and no distant metastasis (M0) are classified as stage 2. Stage 3 is assigned to cancer in which patients have tumors greater than 4 cm in size (T3) or in which there are T1 or T2 tumors and a palpable ipsilateral lymph node less than 3 cm in diameter (N1) and M0. Stage 4 includes cancer in which tumors invade skin or bone (T4) or in which patients have an ipsilateral

Table 3-4 Staging of Esophageal and Pancreatic Cancer

		Pancreas	Esophagus
Tumor			
Tis		—	Carcinoma in situ
T1		—	Involvement of lamina propria
T1a		Limited to pancreas < 2 cm	—
T1b		Limited to pancreas > 2 cm	—
T2		Invasion of duodenum, common bile duct, peripancreatic tissues	Invasion of muscularis
T3		Invasion of the stomach, spleen, colon, or blood vessels	Invasion of the adventitia
T4		—	Invasion of adjacent mediastinal structures
Nodes			
N0		No nodal involvement	No nodal involvement
N1		Nodal metastases	Nodal metastases
Metastasis			
M0		None	None
M1		Distant metastases	Distant metastases
Stage Groupings			
	I	T1–2, N0, M0	T1, N0, M0
	II	T3, N0, M0	
	IIA		T2 or T3, N0, M0
	IIB		T1 or T2, N1, M0
	III	T1–3, N1, M0	T4, N0, M0
			T1–3, N1, M0
	IV	Any T, any N, M1	Any T, any N, M1

lymph node greater than 3 cm in size (N2) or bilateral palpable lymph nodes (N2) or the presence of distant metastasis (M1).

Sequential Staging Approach

A complete history and physical examination form the foundation of clinical staging. Routine laboratory tests such as multichannel chemistries and measurement of serum enzyme levels help in determining the extent of disease. Elevated levels of serum enzyme such as alkaline phosphatase, lactic acid dehydrogenase, and serum glutamine transaminase are often the first indicator of liver metastases. An elevated serum calcium and/or an elevated serum alkaline phosphatase level are suggestive of bone metastases. It is on the basis of the physical and laboratory findings that one makes decisions regarding whether to use imaging studies, and, if so, whether they should be radiologic or scintigraphic.

Table 3-5 Staging of Gastric Cancer

Stage	
A	Limited to mucosa
B1	Involvement of gastric wall, no modal metastases
B2	Involvement of gastric serosa, no modal metastases
B3	Involvement of adjacent organs, abdominal wall, no nodal metastases
C1	Nodal metastases, limited to gastric wall
C2	Nodal metastases, invasion of entire gastric wall (serosa)
C3	Nodal metastases, invasion of adjacent organs
D	Distant metastases

Table 3-6 Staging of Lymphoma (Hodgkin and Non-Hodgkin)

Stage	
I	Tumor confined to a single lymph node or a single contiguous lymph node chain above or below the diaphragm
II	Tumor confined to two contiguous lymph nodes or nodal chains above or below the diaphragm
III	Tumor involving lymph node chains above and below the diaphragm
IV	Involvement of parenchymal organs such as bone marrow, liver, pleural space, or multiple sites, such as skin, lung, bone, etc.
Modifiers	A - absence of fever, night sweats, weight loss >10% body weight B - presence of fever, night sweats, weight loss >10% body weight E - extranodal involvement of a single site in skin, thyroid, bone, gastrointestinal tract

Physicians have an array of imaging procedures from which to choose. When making decisions regarding which particular imaging procedure to order, it is best to answer the following questions: What is one trying to achieve—the detection of malignant disease or information regarding its anatomic extent? What is the availability and quality of the specific imaging procedure considered? What is the level of expertise of the radiologist who will interpret the imaging? Another factor to keep in mind is that in clinical

Table 3-7 Sensitivity, Specificity, Positive and Negative Predictive Values and Accuracy

Sensitivity = TP/TP + FN
Specificity = TN/TN + FP
Positive Predictive Value = TP/TP + FP
Negative Predictive Value = TN/TN + FN
Accuracy = TP + TN/TP + FP + TN + FN

FN = false negative; FP = false positive; TN = true negative; TP = true positive.

Table 3-8 Staging Work-up for Malignancies

Cancer	Staging Work-up
Head and neck cancer	CXR, CT of neck, panendoscopy
Lung cancer	CXR, upper endoscopy, barium swallow, CT of chest and abdomen
Esophageal cancer	CXR, upper endoscopy, barium swallow, CT of chest and abdomen
Breast cancer	Mammography, chest radiography, axillary lymph node/sentinel node biopsies
Gastric cancer	CXR, UGI, gastroscopy/duodenoscopy, abdominal CT
Pancreatic cancer	CXR, abdominal CT
Colonic cancer	CXR, colonoscopy, barium enema, abdominal CT
Rectal cancer	CXR, abdominal and pelvic CT, transrectal ultrasonography
Bladder cancer	CXR, cystoscopy, pelvic CT
Prostate cancer	CXR, PSA, transrectal prostate ultrasonography, pelvic CT, bone scan
Renal cancer	CXR, IVP, abdominal and pelvic CT, possible MRI, angiography
Ovarian cancer	CXR, endovaginal ultrasonography, abdominal and pelvic CT, barium enema
Endometrial cancer	CXR, endovaginal ultrasonography, abdominal and pelvic CT
Cervical cancer	CXR, endovaginal ultrasonography, abdominal and pelvic CT
Lymphoma	CXR, CT (chest, abdomen, pelvis), possible PET, bone marrow aspirate + core biopsies
Testis cancer	CXR, abdominal and pelvic CT of abdomen + pelvis, possible PET

CXR = chest radiography; CT = computed tomography; UGI = upper gastrointestinal series; PSA = prostate-specific antigen; IVP = intravenous pyelography; MRI = magnetic resonance imaging; PET = positron emission tomography.

medicine there is a spectrum of possible findings with any imaging procedure. Although many times we tend to think of imaging findings as binary—positive or negative—the fact is that more than two outcomes are possible. There are in fact five possible outcomes: positive, probably positive, equivocal, probably negative, and negative. Yet despite the fact that there are five outcomes, the sensitivity, specificity, positive predictive value, negative predictive value, and accuracy are based on binary outcomes (Table 3-7). In this section, we review imaging procedures and their potential roles in defining the extent of disease. The staging procedures for many of the common malignancies are summarized in Table 3-8.

Imaging of the Breast

In response to the prevalence of breast cancer in the United States and the heightened public awareness of this disease as a health care problem, attempts are being made to decrease mortality through early detection. Mammography is important as a screening tool that allows for early detection of cancer. In addition, mammography is a valuable diagnostic tool for women with a dominant breast mass. The two types of mammographic procedures are screening mammography and diagnostic mammography.

Screening Mammography

Screening mammography is the best way to diagnose a clinically occult breast cancer. Although the age at which women should begin screening mammography has been the subject of debate, there is now consensus that screening mammography should begin at age 40 years and should be done yearly. The views that are obtained of the breast in the screening mammogram are the mediolateral oblique (MLO) (Fig. 3-1) and the cranial-caudal (CC) views (Fig. 3-2). The MLO is the most effective single view and images most of the breast, including the upper-outer quadrant and the axillary tail.

Diagnostic Mammography

Diagnostic mammography or a dedicated mammogram is indicated when there are clinical findings such as a palpable "lump" or "lumps" or abnormal findings on screening mammography that require additional imaging. Diagnostic mammography is a complete work-up tailored to a specific clinical problem and includes views of the breast through the use of spot compression, magnification, and breast ultrasonography. Diagnostic mammography should be performed in women older than 30 years when a biopsy is being

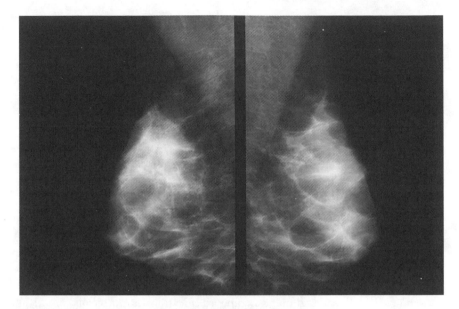

Figure 3-1 A normal mammogram: mediolateral oblique view.

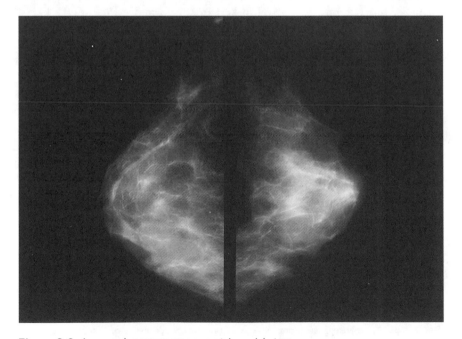

Figure 3-2 A normal mammogram: cranial-caudal view.

planned. Diagnostic mammography is indicated when the lesion in question needs to be better defined and when any unexpected, clinically occult tumors, such as intraductal carcinoma or multifocal breast cancers, need to be defined. In an attempt to help standardize the reporting of mammographic abnormalities, the American College of Radiology Section on Breast Imaging Data and Reporting has suggested the categorization of mammographic abnormalities as shown in Table 3-9.

By using standard terminology in reporting the results of mammography, the treating physician will be less confused about what the mammographic abnormalities represent. Using a standard terminology also allows for better comparability of data.

Mammographic Abnormalities

Mammographic abnormalities include malignant masses (Fig. 3-3) that have ill-defined or spiculated margins and malignant calcifications that are typically numerous, clustered, heterogenous in size and shape, and linear and/or branching. The linear and/or branching calcifications are typically found in the comedo type of DCIS and form the necrotic center. In DCIS noncomedo type, the calcifications vary in size and shape as they lodge within the cribriform spaces within the breast duct. Subtle findings include an asymmetry in the breast parenchyma (Fig. 3-4). Marked architectural distortion of the breast parenchyma heightens the probability of breast cancer, and a biopsy is indicated in these patients.

Breast Ultrasonography

Breast ultrasonography should not be used for screening. Breast ultrasonography is an important adjunct to mammography and is used to characterize palpable abnormalities or to clarify equivocal mammographic findings. It is also used to guide cyst aspirations and needle biopsies. Ultrasonography can dis-

Table 3-9 Assessment Categories of Mammography (Standard Terminology as Recommended by the American College of Radiology)

Category	Assessment	Descriptor
I	Negative	
2	Benign finding	Benign abnormality
3	Probably benign	High probability; short-term follow up
4	Suspicious abnormality	Possibly benign finding; suspicion of cancer; biopsy should be considered
5	Highly suggestive of cancer	Abnormality suggestive of cancer; action should be taken

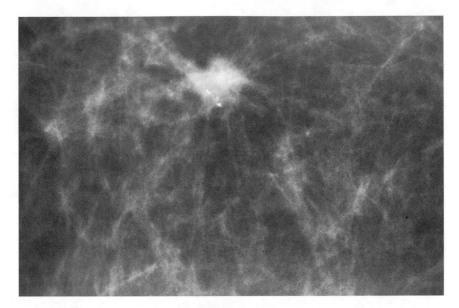

Figure 3-3 An abnormal mammogram showing a small mass with microcalcifications. A stereotactic biopsy showed an invasive breast cancer. A lumpectomy showed a 5-mm infiltrating ductal carcinoma.

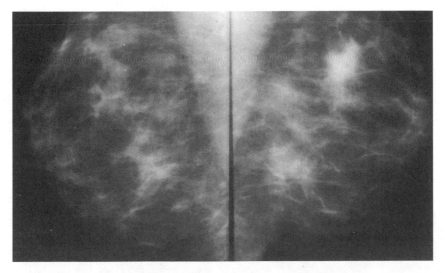

Figure 3-4 An abnormal mammogram demonstrating asymmetrical breast parenchyma in a patient with a palpable mass. The excisional biopsy showed an infiltrating lobular carcinoma.

criminate cystic from solid masses, particularly when they are identifiable only through mammography.

Magnetic Resonance Imaging of the Breast

To date, magnetic resonance imaging (MRI) of the breast has been used to identify rupture of a silicone breast implant (intracapsular or extracapsular). Magnetic resonance imaging with intravenous magnetic resonance contrast agents may have a potential role in detecting breast cancer. In the future, potential roles of MRI include evaluating suspicious mammographic abnormalities, determining the size and extent of invasive breast cancers, imaging an extremely dense breast, and identifying recurrent breast cancer in an irradiated breast.

Computed Tomography

Computed tomography (CT) measures tissue densities in cross-sectional images in a manner identical to that of conventional radiography, which measures tissue densities in planar images relative to the amount of radiation absorbed by the tissues. However, CT is more sensitive in detecting minor differences in the amount of radiation absorbed by the tissues. Additionally, with CT scans one can peel away layers of tissues and detect small lesions that would be missed or hidden on conventional radiography. The amount of radiation delivered during CT is no more than the amount of radiation used during conventional radiography of the skull, chest, or bone. The use of intravenous iodinated dyes enhances the differences in tissue densities.

Computed tomography has revolutionized the practice of medicine since its introduction almost three decades ago. The use of CT in selected cancers is shown in Table 3-10.

Computed tomography of the chest and upper abdomen to the level of the adrenals are part of the "standard" work-up of lung cancer or suspected lung

Table 3-10 Use of Computed Tomography in Selected Cancers

Tumor	Area Scanned
Head and neck	Neck
Lung	Chest to the adrenals
Esophageal	Chest
Colon, gastric, pancreatic	Abdomen
Kidney	Abdomen and pelvis
Lymphoma	Chest, abdomen, and pelvis
Rectal	Pelvis
Testis	Abdomen and pelvis
Bladder	Pelvis

cancer. Computed tomography of the chest has a high degree of sensitivity and specificity in detecting hilar lymph nodal involvement—66% and 78%, respectively. Similarly, CT of the chest has a high degree of sensitivity and specificity in detecting mediastinal nodal metastases—79% and 65%, respectively. A patient with lung cancer who has enlarged (>2 cm) ipsilateral (stage IIIA lung cancer) or bilateral (stage IIIB unresectable lung cancer) mediastinal lymph nodes is not a surgical candidate and no any additional staging (i.e., mediastinoscopy) is needed. The rationale for examining the adrenal glands is based on the observation that lung cancers frequently metastasize to this organ. However, one must keep in mind that an occasional patient may have a primary adrenal adenoma that is nonfunctional. As the presence or absence of metastatic involvement very greatly influences the therapeutic approach, one must prove the presence of either a benign lesion or a metastasis. Magnetic resonance imaging of the adrenal glands helps differentiate an adrenal adenoma from a metastatic lesion. Adrenal adenomas have a high signal on the T2-weighted image.

Computed tomography of the chest is indicated for the staging of esophageal cancer. The CT detects the degree of thickening of the esophageal wall and the presence or absence of metastases to mediastinal lymph nodes. Computed tomography of the chest is part of the usual staging procedure for patients with Hodgkin disease and the non-Hodgkin lymphomas.

Abdominal CT is the imaging procedure of choice for examining the liver, kidney, pancreas, adrenals, and the para-aortic lymph nodes. It is preferable to do an uninfused and a dynamic CT with slow intravenous contrast. This is the best procedure for detecting hepatic metastases. Whereas ultrasonography of the liver detects a hepatic metastasis less than 1 cm in only 20% of cases, a dynamic abdominal CT detects a hepatic metastasis less than 1 cm in 49% of cases. Occasionally, a serendipitously discovered low-density lesion is detected in the liver on the abdominal CT scan. The average incidence is 17%. A single lesion may represent a cavernous hemangioma. Additional testing is required to document the presence of either a solitary metastatic lesion or a hepatoma or hemangioma. Magnetic resonance imaging of the liver or a nuclear medicine ^{99m}Tc red blood cell scan is helpful in documenting the presence of a hemangioma.

Abdominal CT is the procedure of choice in the staging of a known pancreatic cancer or in the work-up of a suspected pancreatic cancer. Abdominal CT is part of the initial work-up of renal cell cancer and can detect extracapsular penetration and/or para-aortic lymph node involvement. Magnetic resonance imaging of the kidney is more sensitive than CT in detecting thrombus in the renal vein (see section on MRI, p 58).

Computed tomography of the pelvis plays a role in the staging of bladder cancer. Pelvic CT can detect enlarged pelvic lymph nodes. When the bladder is filled with air, CT provides information on the thickness of the bladder wall and any adjacent organ infiltration. Pelvic CT coupled with abdominal CT is used in the staging of rectal cancer.

Magnetic Resonance Imaging

The principle of MRI is the induction of a magnetic field that is strong enough to pull hydrogen atoms away from their axis. This is done through a short burst of radio waves. When hydrogen atoms are deflected from their axis, they emit radio waves at their resonant frequency. These radio waves are in turn picked up by external radio wave detectors that then compute an image (map) of the hydrogen atom radio wave emissions.

Magnetic resonance imaging of the brain is more detailed and more sensitive than CT of the brain; therefore, for imaging the brain, MRI is preferred. Additionally, MRI of the long bones and the axial skeleton is preferable to CT. Magnetic resonance imaging of the bone can provide more detail and can pick up relatively small metastases that might otherwise be missed by CT. Furthermore, MRI of a vertebral body or the pelvis can detect alterations in the bone marrow space. (The role of MRI of the breast is discussed earlier in this chapter.)

Ultrasonography

Because most cancer staging is done with CT, the role of ultrasonography in staging is relatively limited. At present, abdominal ultrasonography is considered only an adjunct to abdominal CT, whereas CT is the preferred method for evaluating hepatic metastases and hepatoma. Alternatively, abdominal ultrasonography of the hepatic biliary system and common bile duct is the preferred imaging procedure in patients with jaundice. Abdominal ultrasonography can readily distinguish intrahepatic from extrahepatic obstruction.

The other roles of ultrasonography include the initial evaluation of pelvic masses and imaging of the prostate, rectum, and testicles. Ultrasonography of the pelvis is the first choice for the evaluation of suspected pelvic masses. More recently, the use of endovaginal ultrasonography produces high-quality images of the uterus and ovaries and is preferred to transabdominal pelvic ultrasonography. In women who are at high risk for ovarian cancer or who are nulliparous, endovaginal ultrasonography is a useful screening procedure.

Transrectal ultrasonography can be used to image the prostate in men who have a palpable prostatic nodule or nodules or men with an elevated level of prostate-specific antigen. The information gleaned by prostatic ultrasonography coupled with measurement of the serum PSA can help determine the stage of prostate cancer.

Transrectal ultrasonography is also useful in determining the depth of penetration of a rectal cancer. Testicular ultrasonography is helpful in distinguishing cystic from solid testicular masses.

Radionuclide Imaging

Radionuclide imaging has been among the oldest forms of imaging in clinical oncology. Long before the advent of computed tomography as a method of detecting hepatic metastases, clinicians would use technetium-99m (^{99m}Tc) liver-spleen scanning for this purpose. The earliest form of radionuclide imaging was the use of iodine isotopes to image the thyroid and treat thyroid carcinomas. Over the past 5 years, significant advances in nuclear medicine have taken place along three parallel tracts: (1) advances in radiochemistry; (2) newer imaging methods; and (3) the use of monoclonal antibodies or monoclonal antibody fragments.

The advances in radiochemistry and gamma camera software and hardware have led to the widespread application of single photon emission computed tomography (SPECT). Developments in radiochemistry have also resulted in the use of ^{18}F, ^{13}N, and ^{11}C positron emitting isotopes in positron emission tomography. The development of monoclonal antibodies to carcinoembryonic antigen, small cell lung cancer antigens, ovarian cancer antigens, and the somatostatin receptor have led to imaging techniques with radiolabeled monoclonal antibodies or antibody fragments. In the future, as the number of monoclonal antibodies against still more specific antigens or receptors increases, we are likely to see even more sophisticated imaging techniques.

Bone Scintigraphy

Bone scintigraphy is performed with technetium–99m (^{99m}Tc) pyrophosphate. The principle of bone scanning is based on the fact that metastatic tumors to bone provoke an osteoblastic response. The ^{99m}Tc pyrophosphate that is used as the scanning agent is laid down in the new bone formed with the ^{99m}Tc incorporated in the hydroxyapatite crystal. The ^{99m}Tc incorporated is detected by the gamma camera. Areas of uptake are indicative of metastatic involvement. Bone scanning is quite sensitive in detecting metastatic involvement (88% sensitivity and 92% specificity). The true-positive rate is 96%, and the true-negative rate is 97%. Bone scanning is an excellent means of detecting bone metastases, doing so long before conventional radiography is able to show lytic or blastic changes. Bone scanning is not indicated in multiple myeloma because the osteoblastic response to myeloma is diminished or nonexistent; therefore, the results of bone scanning in patients with myeloma are usually normal. A situation in which the results of bone scanning may be falsely positive is trauma to the rib cage. A single lesion in a rib or multiple lesions in a linear distribution found on bone scanning are more likely to be traumatic rather than metastatic (Fig. 3-5).

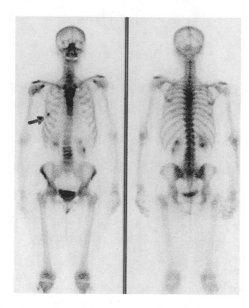

Figure 3-5 ^{99m}Tc bone scan in a patient with stage II breast cancer. The patient complained of low back pain that prompted the current bone scan. The thoracic and lumbar areas showed mild degenerative changes. The single area of uptake in the right seventh rib was related to trauma. The patient recalled bumping the right side of her chest during a bicycling accident earlier that month.

Although bone scanning is highly sensitive in detecting bone metastases, it is not particularly useful in determining response to therapy. A patient who is responding to therapy and who has bone lesions that are healing may show a "flare" phenomenon on bone scanning. This flare phenomenon, or "pseudo-progression," is related to osteoblasts' laying down new bone in a formerly lytic lesion. Bone scans in patients responding to therapy may remain unchanged for months.

Gallium-67 Scintigraphy

Gallium-67 citrate (^{67}Ga) scintigraphy has a role in evaluating patients with malignant lymphoma, particularly in the setting of Hodgkin disease and malignant lymphoma (follicular or diffuse large cell type). Gallium-67 citrate binds to transferrin, and the gallium-67 transferrin complex is bound by transferrin receptors expressed on rapidly growing tumor cells. The gallium-67 citrate transferrin complex will not be bound if the transferrin receptor is down-regulated, as occurs with steroids (a false-negative result). Gallium scanning is most helpful in patients with Hodgkin disease or large cell lymphoma with mediastinal masses. In both settings, a residual smaller mediastinal mass may be present after the completion of therapy. This residual mediastinal mass may represent nothing more than fibrous connective tissue. In this clinical setting, gallium scanning can differentiate the presence of disease (uptake in the mediastinum) from fibrosis (no mediastinal uptake).

Positron Emission Tomography

Positron emission tomography (PET) is a scintigraphic method that creates high-resolution three-dimensional tomographic images of the distribution of the positron-emitting radionuclides in the human body. The radionuclides used include substrates, ligands, drugs, antibodies, neurotransmitters, and other biologic molecules that are utilized for specific biologic processes. The resultant image is that of the specific biochemical or physiologic processes. The positrons used in PET and the half-lives are shown in Table 3-11.

Early in the use of PET, studies were initially focused on the physiology of the brain and heart. More recently, increasing focus has been on PET studies in cancer. Cellular transformation to a malignant phenotype is accompanied with subtle but fundamental changes in metabolism (an increase in DNA synthesis, amino acid uptake, and glycolysis). The increase in glycolysis associated with the malignant phenotype is not a new observation; Warburg reported this observation in the 1930s. Fluorodeoxyglucose (FDG) is a tracer of glycolysis. FDG is distributed within the blood and is actively taken up within a cell by an active transmembrane, noninsulin-dependent, transport protein called Glut-I. Once FDG is intracellular, the enzyme hexokinase phosphorylates FDG. Once phosphorylated, FDG-6-phosphate is not a suitable substrate for glucose-6-isomerase and FDG-6-phosphate continues to accumulate intracellularly for as long it is being transported. The only way for FDG-6-phosphate to leave its intracellular compartment is via the phosphorylase enzyme, which can convert FDG-6-phosphate to FDG, which in turn can then exit via the Glut-I transport protein. The rate-limiting step in the transport and retention of glucose in most tissues is the ratio of hexokinase/phos-

Table 3-11 Radiotracers Used in Positron Emission Tomography

Atom	Half-life	Radiation Decay
Oxygen-15	123 sec	Beta 1.7 MeV
Nitrogen-13	10 min	Beta 1.2 MeV
Carbon-11	20 min	Beta 0.97 MeV
Fluorine-18	110 min	Beta 0.63 MeV
Iodine-124	4.15 d	Beta 2.4 MeV and gamma

phorylase. In tissues that undergo active glycolysis, such as malignant tumors, brain, and the heart, FDG-6-phosphate remains trapped within these tissues because the ratio of hexokinase/phosphorylase is high, and this represents a metabolic trap for FDG. By labeling FDG with F-18, 18-FDG is an excellent imaging agent to be used in PET.

Positron emission tomography with 18-FDG is dependent on tissue oxygenation, blood flow, peritumoral inflammatory reactions. In inflammatory states, especially in granulomatous diseases, sarcoid, and abscess formation, the results of 18-FDG PET scanning are positive. Although 18-FDG PET scanning is an extremely sensitive technique, one must use careful patient selection and rigorous correlation with other imaging modalities to minimize false-positive and false-negative results.

The indications for FDG PET are listed in Table 3-12. FDG PET is an excellent imaging modality in the work-up of a solitary pulmonary nodule with an excellent degree of diagnostic accuracy (positive predictive value, 94%; negative predictive value, 100%). Given the negative predictive value, a solitary pulmonary nodule that has no uptake on FDG PET is certainly benign. Preliminary data suggest that FDG PET may have a role in differentiating questionable lesions on mammography. Also, FDG PET is a superior means of accessing hilar and mediastinal lymph nodes (sensitivity, 85%; specificity, 81%; positive predictive value, 85%; negative predictive value, 81%). Its diagnostic accuracy is better than that of chest CT, which has a sensitivity of 64%, specificity of 68%, a positive predictive value of 67%, and a negative predictive value of 65%.

Similarly, in women with breast cancer, preliminary studies suggest that FDG PET has a high degree of sensitivity and specificity for the tumor in the

Table 3-12 Clinical Indications for Fluorodeoxyglucose Positron Emission Tomography

Differential Diagnosis
  Solitary pulmonary nodule
  Pancreatic masses
  Breast cancer
Preoperative Staging
  Lung cancer
  Esophageal cancer
  Colorectal cancer
  Breast cancer
  Melanoma
  Sarcoma
  Lymphoma
Differentiation of fibrosis versus residual disease
Suspected recurrences
Follow-up of therapy

breast (95% and 100%, respectively) and for axillary lymph nodes (75% and 90%, respectively). Further studies remain to be done to confirm these results with FDG PET in breast cancer; however, if these preliminary findings are correct, FDG PET may obviate the need for axillary dissection and sentinel node biopsy (see Chapter 12).

The role of FDG PET in the preoperative staging of esophageal, colorectal, melanoma, and soft tissue sarcomas continues to emerge. Preliminary data show a high degree of sensitivity and specificity. Additional data and comparative studies are required.

FDG PET has been compared with CT in patients with non-Hodgkin lymphoma. The two comparative trials published included small numbers of patients. Both trials demonstrated that FDG PET identifies more lesions than are demonstrated by CT; however, FDG PET's identification of more areas of involvement did not alter the clinical stage as determined by CT. A potential role for FDG PET in patients with non-Hodgkin lymphoma is in the detection of residual disease and in helping to clarify the presence of residual disease in residual masses in patients who have otherwise achieved a complete response to therapy. Another role for FDG PET is in distinguishing intracerebral lymphoma from central nervous systmem (CNS) toxoplasmosis in patients with acquired immunodefiiciency syndrome (AIDS). Patients with AIDS and CNS lymphoma have intense uptake as identified by FDG PET, whereas those with CNS toxoplasmosis do not.

Pathologic Staging

Pathologic staging is an important aspect of the overall staging process because it provides additional information in making treatment decisions.

Thoracentesis

A patient with a right hilar mass and an ipsilateral effusion may have either an operable lung cancer (if the effusion is the result of right-middle or lower lobe atelectasis) or inoperable lung cancer (if the effusion is malignant). In this setting, a thoracentesis is mandatory in helping one to make the appropriate treatment decision. Similarly, women with an ovarian mass and right-sided pleural effusion may have either Meigs syndrome (pleural effusion with ovarian fibroma or ovarian tumors caused by diaphragmatic defects or diaphragmatic lymphatic channels) or stage IV ovarian cancer. Again, a thoracentesis is required to determine the extent of disease.

I prefer to perform a diagnostic thoracentesis under ultrasonographic guidance. This minimizes the risk of pneumothorax and allows even a small pleural effusion to be approached. In addition, I prefer using a thoracentesis system with a flexible catheter within the thoracentesis needle (Arrow-Clarke Thoracentesis Kit). Once again, this minimizes the risk of pneumothorax. Once the effusion has been identified, the appropriate intracostal space is localized and the skin and soft tissues are anesthestized with 2% lidocaine. A small nick is made in the now anesthestized skin with the tip of a scalpel blade. This facilitates insertion of the needle. Once the needle is within the pleural space, the Arrow-Clarke kit will show a green indicator in the hollow needle. The flexible intracatheter is then inserted into the pleural space and a small volume of fluid is withdrawn (100–150 mL). The patient is bandaged and then sent for post-thoracentesis inspiration and expiration posterior-anterior chest radiography.

Patients with presumed malignancies and ascites require a paracentesis for documenting the extent of disease. The procedure I use is similar to a thoracentesis. The patient is placed in the supine position and the right lower quadrant is chosen. I avoid the left lower quadrant in order to avoid hitting the sigmoid colon. The same tray is used as for a thoracentesis. This allows placement of a flexible silastic catheter in the abdominal space and avoids leaving a metal needle that can penetrate the bowel. The system is a closed one that allows leaving the catheter in place for gravity drainage. Generally 1 to 1.5 L is drained. Patients with ascites are generally volume depleted and should be given some intravenous saline. The volume of saline infused is directly proportional to the quantity of fluid removed if in excess of 1 L so that one avoids hypertension.

Bone Marrow Aspirate and Biopsy

The indications for a bone marrow aspirate and biopsy are listed in Table 3-13. A bone marrow aspirate and biopsy is part of the staging procedure used to help optimize the therapy of patients with Hodgkin disease, non-Hodgkin lymphoma, and small cell lung cancer. Bone marrow aspirate and biopsy are also part of the investigative work-up of any cytopenia. Finally, the procedure helps document the clinical suspicion of an acute myeloid or lymphoid leukemia, chronic myeloid or lymphoid leukemia, or the clinical suspicion of multiple myeloma.

Table 3-13 Indications for Bone Marrow Aspirate and Bone Core Biopsy

Pathologic staging of lymphoma, Hodgkin and non-Hodgkin lymphoma
Pathologic staging of small cell lung cancer
Investigation of cytopenias (thrombocytopenia, anemia, leukopenia, neutropenia)
To confirm the diagnosis of chronic lymphatic leukemia, chronic myeloid leukemia, myeloma, or acute myeloid or lymphoid leukemias

The procedure is relatively straightforward. The patient is placed in the prone position. The iliac wing is carefully palpated until the posterior superior iliac spine is encountered, located usually two fingerbreadths above and two fingerbreadths lateral to the beginning of the gluteal folds. In a thin patient, a slight indentation is present at the site of the posterior iliac spine (Fig. 3-6*A*). This area is then prepped with Betadine or the disinfectant of choice. The skin and muscles are then anesthetized with 2% lidocaine. This generally takes 3 to 5 minutes. After local anesthesia has been achieved, a puncture wound with a scalpel is made and an Illinois Needle® is inserted into the posterior superior iliac spine (Fig. 3-6*B*). Patients should be advised that they will feel a pressure sensation when this is being done. The physician should angle the needle laterally to minimize any possibility of its "falling off" the patient. A 45- to 60-degree angle to the skin is advised. Once the needle has been impaled into the posterior superior iliac spine, the needle should

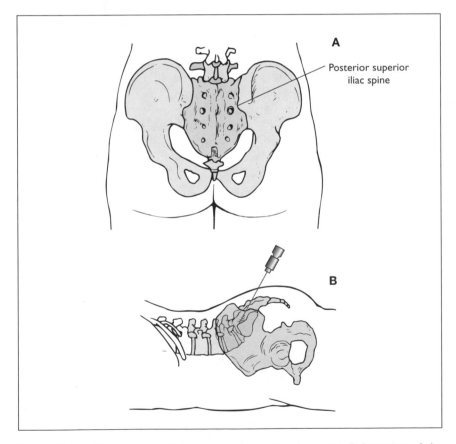

Figure 3-6 *A*, The location of the posterior superior iliac spine. *B*, Insertion of the Illinois Needle® into the posterior superior iliac spine.

be as secure as if imbedded in rock. Any play of the needle is a sign that the needle has not been securely placed. The introducer is removed from the Illinois Needle® (which is hollow) and a 20-mL syringe that has been rinsed with EDTA is inserted into the Leuer-lock of the needle. The EDTA within the syringe complexes the calcium within the blood and thus inhibits the marrow from clotting. It is best to advise the patient at this point that the aspirate procedure will result in a "drawing" pain. A small volume (3–4 mL) of marrow is aspirated. Generally, a technician is present to prepare the aspirate slides. If no technician is available, the physician must prepare his or her own slides. He or she first needs to judge the adequacy of the aspirate *before withdrawing the needle*. To determine if the aspirate is inadequate, the clinician should reintroduce the trocar and quickly squirt a small volume of the marrow onto a glass slide placed at a 45-degree angle (the slides are usually included in the bone marrow aspirate tray) (Fig. 3-7). Blood will run down the slide, and the bone marrow spicules will stick. The bone marrow spicules are yellow-red in color and are tiny (the size of pin-heads). After the blood has run off, the physician should touch the tip of a clean glass slide onto the slide with the spicules. A clean glass slide should then be placed underneath the slide with the adherent spicules on its tip, and the spicules are smeared across the slide. The procedure should be repeated two to three times and these slides be allowed to air dry. The Illinois Needle® should now be removed.

If the bone marrow aspirate yields no spicules or blood, the marrow is "packed" and there is no point in attempting another aspirate. In this case, a bone cell biopsy should be performed. A bone marrow biopsy provides complementary information, and in patients with malignant lymphoma, it is not uncommon for results of the aspirate to be normal and for the biopsy to reveal focal paratrabecular involvement. A bone marrow biopsy should immediately follow the aspirate. The iliac needle is removed, and a Jamshidi needle is inserted in the same puncture wound. The Jamshidi needle is a hollow bone-cutting needle with an internal trocar. The Jamshidi is placed at the same 60-degree angle on top of the posterior superior iliac spine, and in a turn-turn motion, the needle is advanced into the pelvis. The turn-turn motion advances the needle into the bone. The needle turns 30 degrees clockwise and is turned counterclockwise by 30 to 45 degrees while direct pressure is applied to the top of the needle (Fig. 3-8). Again, once the needle is in the bone it should feel like a sword embedded in rock. After it is embedded, the internal trocar is removed and the needle is advanced into the bone for a variable depth (7–15 mm). The lengths of the core can be estimated by replacing the internal trocar. The difficult part is now removing the Jamshidi needle. If it is removed by pulling it straight out, the core will remain in the pelvis. The best method of securing the core is to turn the needle clockwise four to five revolutions and counterclockwise four to five revolutions. The needle should be jiggled two to three times and then removed by being turned counterclock-

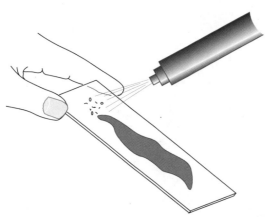

Step 1
With slide tilted at 45°, a few drops of the marrow aspirate are sprayed on the slide and blood is allowed to run down. The marrow particles stick to the top.

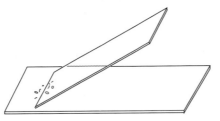

Step 2
With a clean slide, touch the marrow particles to the tip of the clean slide.

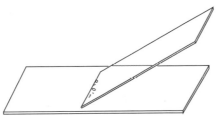

Step 3
Take another clean slide and smear the top of the slide containing the marrow particles across the clean slide.

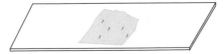

Figure 3-7 Steps involved in making a bone marrow aspirate smear.

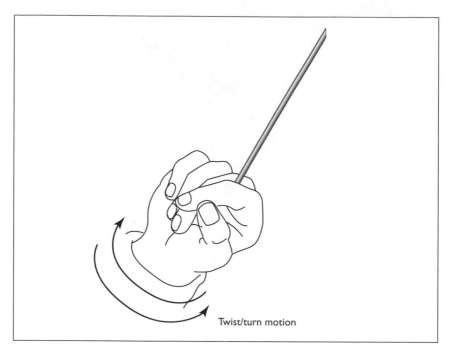

Twist/turn motion

Figure 3-8 The twist-turn motion involved in performing a bone core biopsy.

wise while being withdrawn. The bone core resembles a small portion of a toothpick. It can be rolled on a glass slide to make a bone core touch prep, after which it is placed in formalin.

Mediastinopscopy

Mediastinoscopy is a pathologic staging procedure used in patients with non–small cell lung cancer. It allows the thoracic surgeon to review and inspect the right paratracheal node by making a small incision in the suprasternal notch and inserting a mediastinoscope in the right paratracheal space. A suprasternal mediastinoscopy does not allow access to the left paratracheal nodes because of the aortic arch. A left parasternal mediastinotomy allows access to the left-sided mediastinal nodes. With the advent of FDG PET, the indications for mediastinoscopy and mediastinotomy are becoming fewer. At present, in a patient with suspected or proven non–small cell lung cancer who has mediastinal lymph nodes less than 1 cm on chest CT and no uptake in the mediastinum on PET, it is pointless to proceed with a mediastinoscopy and mediastinotomy. A thoracotomy should be performed. Similarly, if there is obvious mediastinal involvement (mediastinal lymph nodes >2 cm) and up-

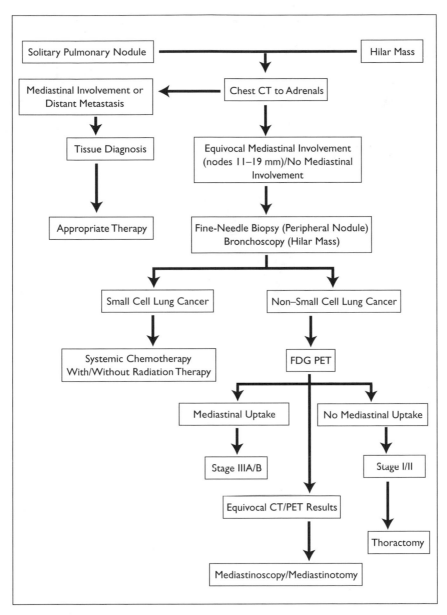

Figure 3-9 The approach to a patient with a solitary pulmonary nodule of hilar mass.

take in the mediastinum on PET, then it is not worthwhile to perform mediastinoscopy and mediastinotomy. Mediastinoscopy is reserved for patients with equivocal findings on either CT or FDG PET (Fig. 3-9).

Chapter 4

Oncologic Emergencies

Superior Vena Obstruction

The superior vena cava (SVC) is a large but thin-walled vein and is easily compressed. The SVC is encircled by lymph node chains that drain all the structures of the right thoracic cavity and the lower part of the left thoracic cavity. When the SVC is partially or completely obstructed, the azygos venous system and other systems, including the internal mammary, lateral thoracic, paraspinous, and the esophageal venous systems, participate in developing a collateral circulation. The malignancies that are etiologically associated with SVC obstruction are lung cancers, both small cell and non–small cell, the non-Hodgkin lymphomas, germ cell tumors of the mediastinum, and thymomas. Hodgkin disease rarely causes SVC obstruction.

Breast cancer is the most common metastatic tumor that results in SVC compression. Nonmalignant causes include central venous catheters, cardiac pacemakers, and mediastinal fibrosis. With the increasing use of central venous catheters in cancer patients, nonmalignant causes of SVC obstruction are likewise increasing.

The symptoms of SVC obstruction are insidious in nature and include dyspnea, facial swelling or fullness, cough, arm swelling, chest pain, and dysphagia (Table 4-1). The physical signs include venous distension of the side or chest wall, facial edema, cyanosis, plethora of the face, and edema of the arms (see Table 4-1).

Although SVC obstruction used to be considered a medical emergency, it simply is not. Conservative measures such as elevation of the upper body and

Table 4-1 Symptoms and Signs of Superior Vena Cava Obstruction

Symptoms	Physical signs
Dyspnea	Venous distention of neck
Facial swelling	Venous distention of chest wall
Head fullness	Facial edema
Cough	Cyanosis
Arm swelling	Plethora of the face
Chest pain	Edema of the arms

head and treatment with diuretics can be carried out to provide symptomatic relief while one investigates the cause. In most instances, the cause is a mediastinal mass, in which case it becomes imperative to establish a histologic diagnosis before treatment is instituted. Performing mediastinal irradiation before a biopsy causes the biopsy to be uninterpretable in half of the patients. The single most useful test is computed tomography of the chest, which provides useful information about the SVC, mediastinum, bronchia, and heart. Venography in the diagnosis of SVC obstruction has a limited role, if any.

Arriving at a histologic diagnosis is the first priority in SVC obstruction because the histologic diagnosis determines the type of treatment to be administered. If a patient has palpable peripheral lymph adenopathy or pleural effusion, these should be investigated first. Biopsy should be done on an enlarged peripheral node (see Chapter 2, pp 24–25, 31). A thoracentesis can be performed. Sputum cytologic testing carries a diagnostic yield of 49%. In the absence of a positive cytologic test result, peripheral adenopathy, or a pleural effusion, procedures that should be done are a mediastinoscopy or a percutaneous transthoracic computed tomography–guided fine-needle biopsy; these procedures yield a histologic diagnosis in 81% to 88% of cases.

Before specific therapy is started, general measures that provide temporary benefits include bed rest; elevation of the head; oxygen to reduce the venous pressure and increase the cardiac output; and diuretics, which reduce the edema and have a great palliative effect. Traditionally, steroids have been used, but they have an as yet unproven role.

The goals of treatment of SVC obstruction are palliation of symptoms and cure, depending on the underlying tumor. For patients with small cell lung cancer and non–small cell lung cancer, chemoradiation or radiation therapy alone may be appropriate treatment (see Chapter 9, pp 159-164). For patients with breast cancer, mediastinal irradiation is an effective mode of palliation. Chemotherapy alone, radiation therapy alone, or chemoradiation therapy are effective modes of treatment for SVC obstruction caused by non-Hodgkin lymphomas.

Catheter-induced SVC obstruction is increasing in frequency. It is caused by a thrombosis within the SVC as a consequence of the central line. When

SVC obstruction is caused by a central line catheter, treatment is to remove the central line and start thrombolytic therapy with either streptokinase, urokinase, or recombinant tissue plasminogen activator *early in the course of the central line thrombosis.* The dose of urokinase is 4000 U/kg over 30 minutes, then 4000 U/kg/h for 24 hours, followed by heparin and the oral anticoagulants.

The dose of streptokinase is 250,000 U over 30 minutes, then 100,000 U/h for 24 hours, followed by heparin and oral anticoagulants. In an established SVC thrombosis of more than 48 hours' duration, treatment with heparin is started and is followed by oral warfarin.

Spinal Cord Compression

Spinal cord or cauda equina compression can complicate the course of patients with cancer. Spinal cord compression (SCC) is truly a medical emergency and overall outcome is most influenced by a patient's neurologic status at the time that treatment is initiated. If one waits for all the physical signs associated with spinal cord or cauda equina compression to develop, it is too late to reverse the neurologic deficit. Patients who receive treatment for SCC while they are still ambulatory remain ambulatory. A general rule to follow is that the development of back pain in a patient with a diagnosis of cancer is SCC until proven otherwise.

Spinal cord or cauda equina compression can result from intradural or extradural metastases. Extradural compression usually results from metastatic involvement to the vertebral body or the neural arch. With vertebral involvement, the metastatic tumor most often compresses the anterior (ventral) aspect of the dural sac. The most common symptom is pain, which is sometimes radicular in nature and is usually increased in intensity with coughing, sneezing, or straining. After a few weeks of persistent pain, symptoms of weakness and then sensory deficits occur. The numbness starts in the toe and ascends. The physical signs include percussion tenderness over the vertebral body, lower extremity weakness, and, late in the course of SCC, a sensory deficit. The cancers most frequently associated with SCC are shown in Table 4-2.

Again, in patients with SCC, treatment is optimized if the diagnosis is made early. My bias is to treat first and investigate later. If I suspect that a patient has SCC based on a history of radicular back pain or pain that increases in intensity with coughing or sneezing, I have the patient immediately begin treatment with high-dose dexamethasone, 4 mg orally every 6 hours, and then I begin the investigation. Radiography of the spine should be first obtained emergently, because in 50% to 60% of patients radiography documents a destructive process. Within hours, radiography should be followed by magnetic resonance imaging or computed tomography (with bone window setting) of

Table 4-2 Cancers Most Frequently Associated with Spinal Cord Compression

Cancer	Frequency (%)
Lung	16
Breast	12
Unknown primary	11
Lymphoma	11
Myeloma	9
Sarcoma	8
Prostate	7
Renal cell	6
Gastrointestinal	4
Thyroid	3
Other	15

Adapted from Bruckman JE, Bloomer WD. Management of spinal cord compression. Semin Oncol. 1978; 5:135–40.

Table 4-3 Factors That Influence Decision Making Regarding the Treatment of Patients with Spinal Cord Compression

Factor	Recommended Treatment
Radiosensitive tumor (e.g., lymphoma, breast, prostate, lung) with no spinal instability	Radiation therapy
Pathologic vertebral fracture *with instability*	Vertebral resection
Radioresistant tumor (e.g., renal cell, sarcoma, unknown primary)	Vertebral resection
Relapse in prior site	Vertebral resection
No response to radiation therapy	Vertebral resection
Relapse after resection or radiation therapy	Chemotherapy
Chemotherapy-sensitive tumor	Chemotherapy

the appropriate area of the spine. These are excellent measures of detecting SCC or cauda equina compression. At present, myelography is seldom used. If there is no evidence of SCC, dexamethasone is discontinued.

After a diagnosis of SCC or caudal equina compression is made, definite treatment is initiated with either radiotherapy alone or surgery (vertebral body resection; laminectomy has led to disappointing results). The factors that help one determine whether to use radiation therapy alone as opposed to surgery and radiation are summarized in Table 4-3.

Although randomized trials have not defined the optimal radiation therapy dose or schedule, usually radiation therapy is administered at a high dose 300 cGy–400 cGy × 3 followed by 150 cGy to a dose that exceeds 2500 cGy. The outcome of therapy is most greatly influenced by the timeliness of the intervention.

Metabolic Emergencies

Patients with cancer may have a variety of metabolic complications, including hypercalcemia, hyperuricemia, tumor lysis syndrome, hypoglycemia, Addison disease, and lactic acidosis (Table 4-4).

Hypercalcemia

Hypercalcemia is the most common metabolic complication in patients with cancer. The cancers most frequently associated with hypercalcemia are listed in Table 4-5. The cause of hypercalcemia in a patient with cancer needs to be explored in the same manner that one explores it in patients without cancer. The physician should not assume it is related to bone metastases, although this is clearly the most frequent cause. Causes of hypercalcemia are listed in Table 4-6; the two most frequent causes of hypercalcemia are primary hyperparathyroidism and cancer. In fact, primary hyperparathyroidism has an increased incidence in women with breast cancer. Thus, careful work-up should be undertaken to determine the exact cause; this investigation includes a calculation of the chloride/phosphate ratio, measurement of serum parathyroid hormone (PTH) level and PTH-related protein level, and, if necessary, urinary cyclic adenosine monophosphate (AMP) (Table 4-7). Patients with hyperparathyroidism usually have asymptomatic hypercalcemia, a chloride/phosphate ratio in excess of 30, an elevated immunoreactive PTH, and a normal or low level of PTH-related protein (Case 4-1). In contrast, patients with malignancy-associated hypercalcemia have a usual chloride/phosphate ratio of less than 30, a normal or low immunoreactive PTH level, and an elevated level of PTH-related proteins.

Table 4-4 Metabolic Complications Associated with Cancer

Hypercalcemia
Hyperuricemia
Tumor lysis syndrome
Hypoglycemia
Addison disease
Lactic acidosis

Table 4-5 Cancers Associated with Hypercalcemia

Breast cancer
Myeloma
Non–small cell lung cancer
Bladder cancer
Prostate cancer

Table 4-6 Causes of Hypercalcemia

Metabolic disorders
  Primary hyperparathyroidism
  Hyperthyroidism
  Pheochromocytoma
  Osteopetrosis

Renal insufficiency
  Secondary hyperparathyroidism

Cancer

Infections
  Tuberculosis
  Human immunodeficiency virus
  Coccidioidomycosis

Sarcoid

Lithium

Dietary excess
  Vitamin D
  Vitamin A
  Milk-alkali

Table 4-7 Laboratory Differences Between Hyperparathyroidism and Hypercalcemia of Malignancy

	Hyperparathyroidism	Hypercalcemia of Malignancy
Serum calcium	▲ Usually >12.5 mg/dL	▲▲ >12.5 mg/dL
Immunoreactive PTH	▲	Normal or low
Chloride/phosphate ratio	>30	<30
PTH-related protein	Normal or low	▲▲
Urinary cAMP	▲	▲

PTH = parathyroid hormone; cAMP = cyclic adenosine monophosphate.
▲ = increased; ▲▲ = markedly increased.

Case 4-1

A 58-year-old woman is seen for a routine follow-up visit for breast cancer. Six years earlier she was diagnosed with stage II breast cancer (T2, N0, M0, ER/PR positive) and had been treated with a modified radical mastectomy and adjuvant tamoxifen for 5 years. The tamoxifen was discontinued 1 year ago. On today's visit her symptoms are lassitude and altered taste. She notes a "salty taste" and therefore has avoided salty foods this past month. The physical findings were entirely unremarkable. A complete blood count (CBC) and a comprehensive metabolic panel (SMAC) are performed. Forty-eight hours later the CBC and SMAC are reviewed.

The CBC was entirely normal; the abnormalities and other relevant electrolytes found on the SMAC are as follows:

Case 4-1—cont'd

Serum Ca	12.9 mg/dL	Serum phosphorus	3.0 mg/dL
Na	140 mEq/L	Alkaline phosphatase	95 U/L
K	4.5 mEq/L		
Cl	112 mEq/L		
CO_2	21 mEq/L		

Based on her laboratory findings and particularly her chloride/phosphate ratio, a tentative diagnosis of hyperparathyroidism is made. A serum PTH measurement, a bone scan, and a urinary cyclic AMP are scheduled. These tests confirm the diagnosis, and she is referred to an endocrinologist for management.

In the past, cancer-related hypercalcemia was believed to be a function of the presence or absence of bone metastases. In patients with bone metastases, the hypercalcemia was believed to be related to bony destruction; in the absence of bone metastases, the hypercalcemia was thought to be related to "ectopic PTH production." Today the prevailing wisdom is that malignancy-related hypercalcemia, even in patients with extensive bone metastasis, is mediated locally by proteins (osteoclast-activating factors and others) produced by malignant cells that lead to bone destruction.

Parathyroid-related protein (PRP) was isolated in the 1980s and has been fully characterized. A great deal of homology exists between PRP and PTH. Parathyroid-related protein is widely distributed, and although its function in normal physiology is unclear, it is widely speculated that it is involved in local signal transduction in bone and is not prevalent in the systemic circulation. Parathyroid-related protein is synthesized at the site of bone metastases. Although PRP does not cause osteoclast activation per se, it does lead to the production of cytokines such as transforming growth factor–alpha, interleukin-1, platelet-derived growth factor, and tumor necrosis factor, which in turn lead to bone resorption. The pathophysiology of how a metastatic tumor in bone leads to bone resorption is quite complex and requires further elucidation.

Nonetheless, the effects of tumor-induced hypercalcemia lead to hypercalcemic nephropathy, which represents focal degenerative change in the renal epithelia, the collecting ducts, distal convoluted tubule, and loop of Henle. Over time renal tubular cell necrosis, interstitial fibrosis, and nephrocalcinosis may result. The most striking defect is an inability to concentrate urine maximally, which leads to polyuria, nocturia, and volume depletion. The symptoms and signs of hypercalcemia include lethargy, polyuria, nocturia, stupor, constipation, and obstipation. This is in part related to fluid loss, which further increases the serum calcium.

Once a diagnosis of cancer-related hypercalcemia is made, it is important to start therapy with vigorous hydration with normal saline at a rate of 200 to 400 mL/h, as dictated by the patient's underlying cardiac status. Traditionally, furosemide is used; however, there are no randomized trials indicating that furosemide and hydration are any better than hydration alone. The severity of the hypercalcemia and the underlying malignancy determine the hypocalcemic therapy to be used, as shown in Table 4-8.

For patients who do not respond to pamidronate, an option is gallium nitrate, which directly inhibits osteoclasts, at a dose of 100 to 200 $mg/m^2/24$ h for 5 days. However, although gallium nitrate is highly effective, it must be given intravenously over 5 days and can lead to nephrotoxicity. Mithramycin, calcitonin, and intravenous etidronate have limited usefulness and are inferior to both pamidronate and gallium nitrate.

Hyperuricemia

Hyperuricemia is uncommon and most often occurs in the setting of hematologic malignancies and bulky disease, such as malignant lymphomas, chronic myelogenous leukemia, chronic lymphocytic leukemia, and extreme leukocytosis. Clinical manifestations include gout, renal insufficiency, and acute renal failure. Obviously, it is acute renal failure that one wants to avoid. The best way to avoid hyperuricemia is to start treatment with allopurinol 300 to 600 mg/d, 1 to 2 days before any cytotoxic therapy is begun, and to discontinue any drugs that increase the serum uric acid levels, such as thiazide diuretics and salicylates. The urine should be kept at a pH of 7.0 or greater with sodium bicarbonate. Aceta-

Table 4-8 Management of Malignancy-Induced Hypercalcemia

Serum Calcium <12 mg/dL	Serum Calcium >12 mg/dL
For lymphoma, myeloma Start prednisone 1–2 mg/kg/d (onset of action 3–5 d) and start treatment for lymphoma/myeloma	Start IV hydration with saline 200–400 mL/h Furosemide 20–40 mg IV q2–4 h until urine output >150–200 mL/h Pamidronate 90 mg IVPB at 1 mg/min (onset of action 24–48 h; efficacy 70%–100%)
For all other cancers Begin treatment of malignancy Etidronate 5–10 mg/kg/d PO and closely monitor renal function	Start treatment of malignancy **Long-term outpatient therapy** Prednisone 1–2 mg/kg/d for lymphoma/myeloma Etidronate 5–10 mg/kg/d for all other cancers

zolamide, a carbonic anhydrase inhibitor, can be used to alkalinize the urine.

Patients who develop hyperuricemia and either acute renal insufficiency or renal failure may require dialysis.

Tumor Lysis Syndrome

Tumor lysis syndrome is the development of hyperuricemia, hyperkalemia, hyperphosphatemia, and hypocalcemia as a result of a rapid malignant cell death with the release of intracellular contents into the bloodstream. Tumor lysis syndrome is a potentially life-threatening and lethal complication of chemotherapy; however, the syndrome is not limited to chemotherapy alone, but also has been described with interferon, tamoxifen citrate, and estrogen therapy for prostate cancer. The syndrome occurs most often in the setting of large tumor burdens, high proliferative fractions that are highly sensitive to chemotherapy such as high-grade lymphoma, leukemia with hyperleukocytosis, and, occasionally, solid tumors such as germ cell tumors or small cell lung cancer.

The best management of tumor lysis syndrome is prevention. Prevention requires assessing the risk. Patients believed to be at risk, such as those with large tumor burdens, should be hydrated before chemotherapy. Allopurinol should be administered before chemotherapy. Sodium bicarbonate should be administered intravenously to alkalinize the urine, despite an absence of evidence that this is effective. If tumor lysis occurs in spite of these preventative measures, it is important to recognize it and treat it. Treatment involves correcting the electrolyte abnormalities, and in the face of worsening renal failure, dialysis should be considered.

Lactic Acidosis

Lactic acidosis is a rare but potentially lethal complication in patients with malignancy. Lactic acidosis is subdivided into type A, which is caused by poor oxygen delivery to peripheral tissues (shock, sepsis), and type B, which is caused by a variety of diseases, such as cancer, renal failure, diabetes, liver disease, and drugs (e.g., metformin). Lactate, a metabolite of pyruvate, is produced in a reaction catalyzed by lactic dehydrogenase and nicotinamide adenine dinucleotide (NAD). If NAD is depleted, gluconeogenesis stops, pyruvate increases, and the anaerobic metabolism of pyruvate to lactate is increased.

Lactic acidosis typically occurs in patients with progressive leukemia or lymphoma. Usually, patients present with hyperventilation and hypotension. The prognosis of patients with cancer and lactic acidosis is quite poor.

Hypoglycemia

Hypoglycemia is a rare complication of malignancy and most frequently occurs in patients with either insulin-secreting islet tumors of the pancreas (insulinoma) or retroperitoneal mesenchymal malignancies such as fibrosarcoma, leiomyosarcoma, rhabdomyosarcoma, and liposarcoma. The pathophysiology of hypoglycemia is the unregulated production of insulin (insulinomas), insulin-like proteins (retroperitoneal sarcomas), or extensive glucose metabolism (retroperitoneal sarcomas) coupled with the failure of regulatory mechanisms that mitigate against hypoglycemia.

Symptoms of hypoglycemia include weakness, dizziness, hunger, confusion, headache, instability, agitation, and combativeness. The physical signs include tachycardia, diaphoresis, pallor, lethargy, seizures, and coma. The diagnosis of hypoglycemia is based on Whipple's triad:

1. Symptoms consistent with hypoglycemia
2. Low plasma glucose concentration
3. Relief of symptoms when glucose levels are normalized

For patients with insulinoma, a fast is conducted and serial glucose, insulin, and C-peptide levels are drawn. In patients with insulinomas, both the insulin and C-peptide levels are elevated.

The treatment of hypoglycemia consists of either intravenous dextrose or, in instances of significant hypoglycemia, glucagon. The most effective management is treating the underlying malignancy.

Adrenal Failure

Although metastases to the adrenal glands are commonly observed in patients with cancer, particularly in those with lung cancer, adrenal insufficiency is rare. Most commonly adrenal insufficiency is iatrogenic and secondary to cyclic steroid administrations. The symptoms or signs of adrenal insufficiency are lassitude, fatigue, hypotension, and hypokalemia.

Physicians should suspect adrenal insufficiency particularly in patients with cancer who have been receiving cyclic steroids. Such patients are predisposed to adrenal insufficiency, especially if they develop neutropenic fever. In such instances, steroid replacement therapy is advised (hydrocortisone sulfate, 100 mg intravenously every 8 hours or an equivalent dosage of an oral steroid).

Obstruction of Ureters

Obstruction of one or both ureters can complicate the course of patients with cancer. The obstruction may be secondary to direct tumor invasion (cervical, bladder, prostate cancer), compression or invasion of both ureters by retroperitoneal or pelvic lymph nodes involved by metastases (lymphoma, gastric cancer, retroperitoneal sarcomas), or metastasis to the ureter (breast cancer). Ureteral obstruction may also occur as a consequence of retroperitoneal fibrosis from surgery, radiation, or chemotherapy.

Acute obstruction of one or both ureters causes colicky flank pain typical of urolithiasis. Chronic unilateral ureteral obstruction provokes no symptoms. Chronic bilateral obstruction is associated with a dull flank ache, diminished urinary output, edema, hypertension, and, eventually, symptoms and signs of uremia. Serum chemistries typically show a chronic metabolic acidosis, renal insufficiency, and hyperkalemia (type IV, renal tubular acidosis).

Treatment of ureteral obstruction actually can be carried out with placement of computed tomography–guided percutaneous nephrostomy tubes (closed procedure) followed by endourologic placement of ureteral stents. The stents can be placed either retrograde by a urologist or antegrade by an invasive radiologist. The type of percutaneous stents used today is made of polyurethane, a flexible material that makes changing of stents easy and causes less encrustation.

Hemorrhagic Cystitis

Hemorrhagic cystitis is the development of diffuse bladder inflammation and hemorrhage usually secondary to the use of chemotherapeutic agents and, rarely, to radiation therapy or viruses. Most commonly, hemorrhagic cystitis is observed in patients undergoing bone marrow transplantation and is usually associated with high-dose cyclophosphamide or ifosfamide. The hepatic metabolites of cyclophosphamide and ifosfamide are phosphoramide mustard and acrolein. Acrolein is the metabolite responsible for hemorrhagic cystitis. Oral cumulative doses of cyclophosphamide in excess of 90 g or a mean cumulative intravenous dose of 18 g puts patients at risk for hemorrhagic cystitis. The symptoms of hemorrhagic cystitis are dysuria and urinary frequency. The laboratory findings show either gross or microscopic hematuria. Fortunately, in most patients with hemorrhagic cystitis, whether it is secondary to drug or radiation therapy or viral infection, do not have serious bladder hemorrhage. Only 20% of patients with cyclophosphamide-induced hemorrhagic cystitis require transfusion. The treatment of hemorrhagic cystitis is conservative management and includes bladder irrigation and cystoscopy with intravascular fulguration. On rare occasions when bleeding cannot be controlled with conservative measures, intravascular instillation of formalin (usually 2% or 4%) is necessary. Prostaglandin E_2 and F_2 have been tried in pilot studies (1,2) and have been reported to be successful.

REFERENCES

1. **Shurafa M, Shumaker E, Cronin S.** Prostaglandin F_2-alpha bladder irrigation for control of intractable cyclophosphamide-induced hemorrhagic cystitis. J Urol. 1987; 137:1230.

2. **Mohiuddin J, Prentice HG, Schey S, et al.** Treatment of cyclophosphamide-induced cystitis with prostaglandin E_2 [Letter]. Ann Intern Med. 1984;101:142.

Chapter 5

Supportive Care

Many of the chemotherapeutic agents used in the treatment of cancer have a narrow therapeutic index. Toxicities of chemotherapy are particularly worrisome. This is also true of radiation therapy; normal tissue toxicities limit the total doses that can be safely administered. The most common reason for hospital admissions among patients with cancer is neutropenic fever, and the second most common reason is toxicities caused by treatment. In this chapter, we review the approach to patients with neutropenic fever, appropriate use of hematopoietic growth factors and antiemetics, the indications for transfusions, and the management of radiation therapy–induced toxicities.

Febrile Neutropenia

Bacterial infections pose a clear-cut risk to patients who are neutropenic (absolute neutrophil count <500 cells/µL). The risk is greatest for patients with an absolute neutrophil count of less than 100 cells/µL and for patients with protracted neutropenia. In patients with febrile neutropenia (>38.3 °C), the infections that predominate are those caused by either aerobic gram-negative bacilli (*Escherichia coli*, *Klebsiella pneumoniae*, *Pseudomonas aeruginosa*) or gram-positive cocci (coagulase-negative staphylococci, β-hemolytic streptococci, and *Staphylococcus aureus*). With the increasing prevalence of indwelling central line catheters, gram-positive infections—particularly infection with coagulase-negative staphylococci—have increased in incidence.

Fungal infection, especially infection with *Candida* species (*Candida albicans* and *Candida tropicalis*) and *Aspergillus* species, may also occur in patients with febrile neutropenia. This is particularly true if patients have been receiving broad-spectrum antibiotics or if patients have protracted neutropenia. Less common fungi include *Trichosporon*, *Fusarium*, and *Rhizopus*.

Viral infections with herpes viruses (herpes simplex virus, varicella-zoster, cytomegalovirus, Epstein-Barr virus) and respiratory viruses (adenovirus, respiratory syncytial virus, parainfluenza virus, influenza A + B, rhinovirus) predominate in patients with febrile neutropenia.

Remarkably, patients with febrile neutropenia have no symptoms or physical signs aside from chills, fever, and/or rigors. The absence of neutrophils precludes any type of inflammatory response, and therefore the typical signs of inflammation are absent. Despite the absence of symptoms, however, a careful physical examination should be undertaken, although this should not delay the start of empiric antibiotic therapy. The diagnostic work-up is shown in Table 5-1.

After the diagnostic work-up, empiric antibiotic therapy is started (Table 5-2 and Fig. 5-1). Single-agent antibiotic therapy is appropriate for most patients. Patients with a known allergic reaction to cephalosporins can be adequately covered with cilastatin-imipenem. Monotherapy avoids potential nephrotoxicity; however, the disadvantage of monotherapy is poor coverage of coagulase-negative staphy-

Table 5-1 Diagnostic Work-up of Febrile Neutropenia

Two sets of blood cultures: one from a peripheral vein; one from a central line for bacteria and fungi
Urine culture and urinalysis
Culture of any drainage from catheter exit site
Stool culture for *Clostridium difficile* and other pathogens
Chest radiography

Table 5-2 Empiric Antibiotic Therapy in Febrile Neutropenia

Single-agent therapy
 Cefepime 1 g IVPB q8h
 Ceftazidime 2 g IVPB q8h
 Cilastatin-imipenem 500 mg IVPB q6h
 Meropenem 1 g IVPB q8h

Combination therapy
Tobramycin/gentamicin 2 mg/kg (loading dose), then 1.5 mg/kg IVPB q8h
                             and
Ceftazidime 2 g IVPB q8H
                      or
Piperacillin 3 g IVPB q4h

lococci and methicillin-resistant *S. aureus*. In addition, ceftazidime alone does not provide coverage for anaerobes or enterococci. However, all of the single-agent monotherapy antibiotics provide excellent coverage for *Pseudomonas aeruginosa*. At the present time, combination therapy is seldom used. The advantages to combi-

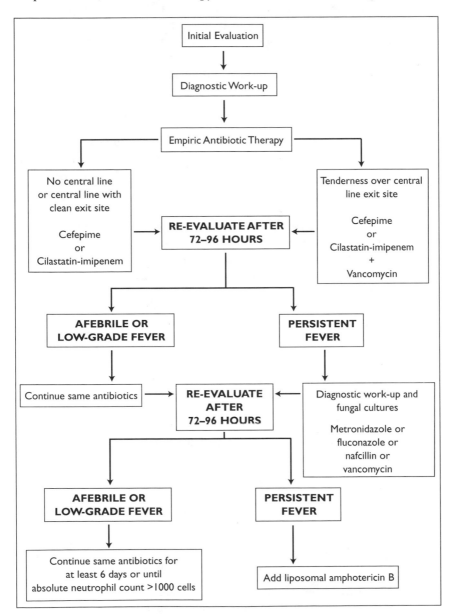

Figure 5-1 An approach to patients with febrile neutropenia.

nation therapy are the possible synergistic effects against gram-negative strains. However, the disadvantages include nephrotoxicity, hypokalemia, and the need to monitor drug levels of the aminoglycoside. These disadvantages outweigh the advantages. Because of the emergence of vancomycin-resistant enterococci, vancomycin is not used as initial empiric therapy for febrile neutropenia. Vancomycin should be considered as part of an initial empiric antibiotic program only if there is evidence of an infection caused by a gram-positive micro-organism (an inflamed central line exit site) and if the prevalence of nosocomial infections caused by methicillin-resistant *S. aureus* is substantial.

Alterations in Initial Empiric Therapy

If after 72 hours of empiric antibiotic therapy the fever begins to abate and a specific organism is identified, antibiotic therapy is modified to optimize the treatment. Antibiotics can be discontinued after 7 days if all evidence of infection is gone and if the patient is no longer neutropenic. If the patient continues to remain neutropenic, antibotic therapy is continued until neutropenia abates.

If fever continues despite 72 to 96 hours of empiric antibiotic therapy, a reassessment is made, the diagnostic work-up is repeated, and changes or additions to the empiric regimen are recommended. Possible changes include:

1. For better gram-positive coverage, adding nafcillin, 2 g intravenously every 4 hours
2. If there is clinical evidence of a potential central line infection, adding vancomycin, 15 mg/kg intravenously every 12 hours
3. For better anaerobic coverage or if there is clinical evidence of typhlitis, adding metronidazole, 500 mg every 6 hours
4. If fungal cultures are positive, adding fluconazole, 400 mg intravenously or orally daily

If fever continues for an additional 96 hours despite these changes, liposomal amphotericin B 5 mg/kg intravenously daily (for the lipid complex) or 3 to 6 mg/kg intravenously daily (for the cholesterol sulfate complex) should be added and fluconazole should be discontinued.

Antiemetics

Considerable progress has been made in the amelioration of chemotherapy-induced nausea and vomiting. Nausea and vomiting is not a natural consequence of chemotherapy administration. With the identification of various serotonin receptors, our understanding of how chemotherapeutics induce nausea and vomiting has improved. It is believed that chemotherapeutic agents produce nausea and vomiting by releasing serotonin from the enterochromaffin cells of the small intestine, and that the released serotonin activates 5-HT_3 receptors (type 3 serotonin receptor) located on the efferents of the vagus nerve to initiate the vomiting

Table 5-3 Emetogenic Potential of Individual Chemotherapeutic Agents*

Emetogenic Potential	Drugs	
High (Level 5) >90% nausea and vomiting	Carmustine Cisplatin >75 mg/m^2 Dacarbazine Thiotepa >200 mg/m^2	Mechlorethamine Melphalan >100 mg/m^2 Streptozocin Cyclophosphamide >1500 mg/m^2
Moderate (Level 4) 60%–90% nausea and vomiting	Carboplatin Ironotecan Cisplatin <50 mg/m^2 Mitoxantrone >14 mg Doxorubicin >60 mg/m^2 Cyclophosphamide >1000 mg/m^2	Ifosfamide Procarbazine Methotrexate >1000 mg Carmustine <250 mg/m^2 Cytarabine >1000 mg/m^2

Mild (Level 3)
30%–60% nausea and vomiting
	Aldesleukin (IL-2)
	Busulfan >4 mg/kg
	Epirubicin
	Daunorubicin
	Mitoxantrone <14 mg
	Hexamethylmelamine
	Methotrexate >25 mg <1000
	  mg
	Cyclophosphamide <750
	  mg/m^2
		Fluorouracil >1000 mg/m^2
		Idarubicin
		Lomustine
		Topotecan
		Cyclophosphamide (PO)
		Doxorubicin <60 mg/m^2

Low (Level 2) 10%–30% nausea and vomiting	Docetaxel Etoposide Gemcitabine Paclitaxel	Methotrexate >50 mg/m^2 Mitomycin C Fluorouracil <1000 mg/m^2 Thiotepa
Minimal (Level 1) <10% nausea and vomiting	Bleomycin Busulfan Chlorambucil Hydroxyurea Fludarabine 2-Chlorodeoxyadenosine	Melphalan (oral) Methotrexate <50 mg/m^2 Thioguanine Vincristine Vinorelbine Vinblastine

*With combinations of chemotherapeutics identify the emetogenicity of each agent: Level 1 agents do not contribute; combinations of Level 2 drugs convert regimen to Level 3; adding Level 3 drugs to Level 3 drugs increases the emetogenicity to Level 4; adding moderate-emetogenicity drugs to Level 3 increases the emetogenicity to Level 5.

Adapted from Hesketh PJ, Kris MG, Grunberg SM, et al. Proposal for classifying the acute emetogenicity of cancer chemotherapy. J Clin Oncol. 1997;15:103-9.

reflex. The serotonin 5-HT$_3$ receptors are located not only on the nerve terminals of the vagus but are also located centrally in the chemoreceptor trigger zone of the area postrema. There are now highly selective antagonists of the 5-HT$_3$ receptor that can ameliorate chemotherapy-induced nausea and vomiting such as ondansetron (Zofran), granisetron (Kytril), and dolasetron mesylate (Anzemet). There are no data that any one of these three 5-HT$_3$ receptor antagonists have differences as to the way in which they bind to the 5-HT$_3$ receptor. Furthermore, once a receptor is bound it remains bound unless displaced by continued serotonin release. Using such highly effective drugs rationally requires that the physician take into account several treatment and patient factors, including the emetogenicity of the chemotherapy used, whether this is the first dose or a subsequent dose of chemotherapy, and whether the nausea and vomiting is acute (occurring within the first 24 hours) or delayed. Definitions of the emetogenicity of chemotherapy are shown in Table 5-3.

The use of the definitions shown in Table 5-3 helps physicians more rationally use the 5-HT$_3$ receptor antagonists, which are expensive and have adverse effects such as headache (granisetron, ondansetron, dolasetron), constipation (granisetron, ondansetron), diarrhea (dolasetron), and fatigue (granisetron, ondansetron, dolasetron).

To prevent acute nausea and vomiting with regimens of moderate or highly emetogenic combinations, any of the 5-HT$_3$ receptor antagonists should be used with intravenous dexamethasone, 10 to 20 mg, as shown in Table 5-4. Such regimens completely abate any nausea or vomiting in 60% to 80% of patients.

Patients on regimens that are mildly emetogenic may be treated with oral ondansetron, 2 mg orally; dolasetron, 100 mg orally; or prochlorperazine, 5 to 10 mg tablets or 15 mg long-acting capsules. Clearly, in this patient subset more comparative trials are required.

Patients on regimens that have low or minimal emetogenicity should receive either prochlorperazine alone or corticosteroids. Patients on regimens with minimal emetogenicity often do not require antiemetics or require prochlorperazine on as-needed basis.

Other phenothiazines have little or no advantage over prochlorperazine. Oral dronabinol (Marinol) is a drug of the past and is now seldom used.

Table 5-4 Treatment Regiments to Prevent Acute Nausea and Vomiting Caused by Moderate to Highly Emetogenic Combinations

Granisetron 32 mg IVPB 30 min before with dexamethasone 10–20 mg IVP
or
Ondansetron 2 mg PO 30 min before with dexamethasone 10–20 mg IVP
or
Dolasetron 100 mg IVP 5–10 min before with dexamethasone 10–20 mg IVP

Delayed Nausea and Vomiting

Nausea and vomiting occurring 24 hours after chemotherapy responds poorly to 5-HT$_3$ antagonists. In this setting, continued use of these agents is expensive and not justified. The mechanism of delayed nausea and vomiting is poorly understood and may in fact be related to 5-HT$_3$ receptor upregulation, altered serotonin release and metabolism, molecular injury to the mucosa cells in the gastrointestinal tract, learned conditioned reflex, or all of these. Decreasing doses of corticosteroids (e.g., prednisone 40 mg/d, 30 mg/d, 20 mg/d × 2 days then discontinue) with lorazepam, 1 mg orally twice daily, seems to diminish delayed nausea and vomiting.

Hematopoietic Growth Factors

The past two decades have witnessed a revolution in molecular biology. This revolution has very tangible benefits, including the production of recombinant human proteins. Over the course of the past decade, a variety of recombinant hematopoietic growth factors, which represent regulatory proteins that play important roles in the growth, survival, and differentiation of blood progenitor cells, have been approved for clinical use. Four recombinant hematopoietic growth factors are currently in clinical use (Table 5-5), and an additional three will shortly be considered for FDA approval (Table 5-6).

Bone Marrow Growth and Differentiation

Over the past two decades, our understanding of bone marrow physiology growth and differentiation has improved. We now know that all bone marrow progenitors arise from a common bone marrow progenitor or stem cell (Fig. 5-2). In humans as well as in murine systems, the bone marrow stem cell has the appearance of a small lymphocyte. It expresses a protein called CD34; it does not express human lymphocyte antigens (HLA); it expresses a low level of c-*kit* receptors, and when stained with rhodamine is dull (CD34$^+$, HLA neg., c-*kit* low, rhodamine dull). Moreover, this cell has the capacity for self-renewal and is able to give rise to long-term hematopoietic colonies in tissue culture. Ultimately, the manner in which stem cells grow and differentiate is under the influence of various hematopoietic growth factors or cytokines that propel uncommitted progenitors to progenitors that commit to the various lineages (see Fig. 5-2). With this basic understanding of bone marrow growth and differentiation, one can begin to see where and why hematopoietic growth factors have clinical relevance.

Table 5-5 Recombinant Hematopoietic Growth Factors in Clinical Use

Growth Factor	Indication
G-CSF (filgrastim [Neupogen])	Myelosuppressive chemotherapy
	BMT for nonmyeloid malignancies
	Severe chronic neutropenia
	Mobilizing bone marrow progenitors for BMT (PBPCs)
GM-CSF (sargramostim [Leukine])	After autologous BMT (administer GM-CSF after BMT delayed engraftment or graft failure)
	After induction chemotherapy for elderly patients with AML
	After allogeneic BMT
	Mobilizing PBPCs
Erythropoietin (Epogen)	Anemia of chronic renal failure
Erythropoietin (Procrit)	Anemia in patients with nonmyeloid malignancies receiving chemotherapy
	Anemia in patients with HIV treated with zidovudine
Interleukin-11 (Neumega)	Chemotherapy-induced thrombocytopenia

BMT = bone marrow transplantation; PBPC = circulating peripheral blood bone marrow progenitor cells; AML = acute myeloid leukemia; HIV = human immunodeficiency virus.

Table 5-6 Hematopoietic Growth Factors in Development

Thrombopoietin
Stem cell factor (c-*kit* ligand)
Interleukin-3/G-CSF fusion protein

Clinical Use of Hematopoietic Growth Factors

Hematopoietic growth factors must be used rationally and optimally because of the high costs associated with their use. The evidence-based guidelines formulated by the American Society of Clinical Oncology (ASCO) are intended to define reasonable use of hematopoietic growth factors and to discourage excess use. Two myeloid growth factors are currently licensed for clinical use in the United States: filgrastim (granulocyte colony-stimulating factor [G-CSF]) and sargramostim (granulocyte-macrophage colony-stimulating factor [GM-CSF]). G-CSF is highly lineage specific and stimulates the production of neutrophils, whereas GM-CSF stimulates the production of neutrophils, monocytes, and eosinophils. Both growth factors have been extensively studied and have FDA-approved indications as shown in Table 5-5. Only one small comparative trial has been conducted comparing GM-CSF with G-CSF (1); based on this trial, the growth factors were deemed equivalent. Both G-CSF and GM-CSF

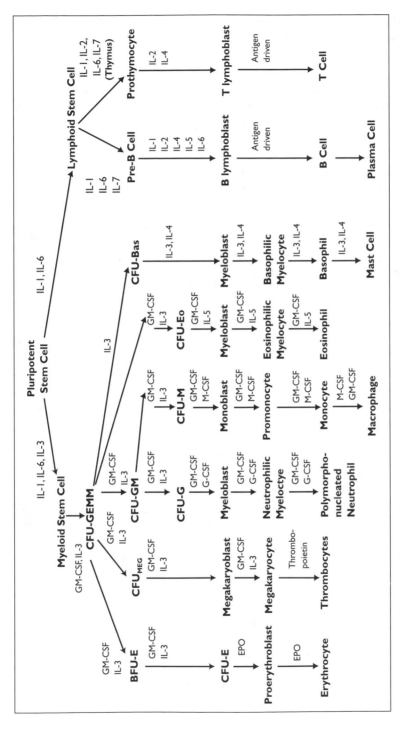

Figure 5-2 Diagram of bone marrow growth and differentiation. All bone marrow progenitors arise from a common stem cell. The subsequent differentiation into the various lineages is governed by cytokines. CFU = colony-forming units; CFU$_{BAS}$ = colony-forming unit–basophil; CFU-E = colony-forming unit—erythroid; CFU-Eo = colony-forming unit—eosinophil; CFU-G = colony-forming unit–granulocyte; CFU-M = colony-forming unit—monocyte/macrophage; CFU$_{MEG}$ = colony-forming unit—megakaryocyte; EPO = erythropoietin; G-CSF = granulocyte colony-stimulating factor; GM-CSF = granulocyte-macrophage colony-stimulating factor; IL = interleukin; M-CSF = macrophage colony-stimulating factor.

are used prophylactically to avoid febrile neutropenia during the first course of chemotherapy, primary prophylaxis, or subsequent courses of chemotherapy in patients who have had an episode of febrile neutropenia (secondary prophylaxis). To use G-CSF or GM-CSF as primary prophylaxis, a chemotherapy regimen must be associated with a high incidence of febrile neutropenia ($\geq40\%$)—that is, a known myelosuppressive regimen. With regimens that are less myelosuppressive, the cost of G-CSF outweighs its potential benefits.

When an episode of febrile neutropenia develops in a patient receiving chemotherapy, it appears prudent to start administering either G-CSF or GM-CSF to avoid recurrent episodes of febrile neutropenia and to continue administering the regimen at the highest possible dose and on schedule.

Both G-CSF and GM-CSF have indications after bone marrow transplantation. Several randomized trials have demonstrated that both G-CSF and GM-CSF at doses of 5 µg/kg can reduce the duration of neutropenia, infections, complications, and the duration of hospitalization after autologous and allogeneic transplantation (2). Both growth factors have proved to be useful in delayed or inadequate neutrophil engraftment after bone marrow transplantation. Over the past decade, there has been an increase in autologous and allogeneic bone marrow transplants in which the progenitor cells are derived from the peripheral blood as opposed to bone marrow (see Fig. 5-2). Both G-CSF and GM-CSF, either alone in high dose (10 µg/kg) or in combination with myelosuppressive chemotherapy (usually cyclophosphamide), can cause the egress of uncommitted and committed bone marrow progenitor cells from the bone marrow cavity into the circulation (mobilization). Although the exact mechanism of this mobilization phenomenon is unknown, it appears that the two growth factors in concert with other cytokines produced in vivo after myelosuppressive chemotherapy alter adhesive proteins that would otherwise anchor uncommitted progenitors (including the true stem cell) to tissue microphages in the marrow cavity that play the role of nutrient cells. Thus, another indication for both G-CSF and GM-CSF is the mobilization of bone marrow progenitors into the peripheral blood (PBPCs) for both autologous and allogeneic bone marrow transplantations.

GM-CSF has been approved for use in elderly patients (>55 years) with acute myeloid leukemias after induction therapy to shorten the time to neutrophil recovery, therefore reducing the potential for severe or fatal life-threatening infections. Trials on the use of GM-CSF in younger patients are ongoing.

Patients with either congenital neutropenia, cyclic neutropenia, or idiopathic neutropenia who have an absolute neutrophil count of less than 500 cells/µL are at risk for recurrent infections and benefit from G-CSF. In this setting, G-CSF normalizes the absolute neutrophil count and reduces the incidence of infection by more than 90%.

G-CSF and GM-CSF are remarkably well tolerated. However, patients can experience toxicities from both (Table 5-7). Both G-CSF and GM-CSF are administered at doses of 5 µg/kg subcutaneously daily, usually after chemotherapy has been completed.

Erythropoietin

Human recombinant erythropoietin (EPO, Epogen, Procrit) is a red cell lineage–specific hormone that stimulates erythrocyte production. Anemia is a common complication of cancer chemotherapy and its presence detracts from quality of life because it typically causes fatigue, exercise intolerance, and, in some cases, depression. Although it is important to determine the cause of anemia in cancer, most often it is multifactorial and related to the diminishment of erythroid progenitors caused by the effects of chemotherapy and/or radiotherapy. Marrow involvement and diminished EPO production as a consequence of inflammatory cytokines such as interleukin-1, tumor necrosis factor, and interferons, which may be elaborated by either the tumor or host defenses, all contribute to the development of anemia. The hypoproliferative anemia caused by diminished EPO production, as consequence of inflammatory cytokines, is the "anemia of chronic disease." Thus, if during the course of chemotherapy the baseline hemoglobin decreases to less than 10.5 g/dL or if a patient with cancer is already anemic, it is reasonable to begin Procrit at an initial dose of 150 U/kg subcutaneously three times per week. If the patient does not respond to Procrit after 4 weeks of therapy, the dose is increased to 300 U/kg subcutaneously three times per week. More recently, an alternative dosing regimen of 40,000 U/mL once per week appears to be as efficacious as the three times per week dosing schedule. The dose of Procrit is titrated downward or the frequency is decreased to one to two times per week after the hematocrit is in excess of 40%. EPO is extremely well tolerated; its adverse effects are diarrhea, edema, and in cancer patients (rarely) hypertension or seizures.

Table 5-7 Toxicities of Filgrastim (G-CSF) and Sargramostim (GM-CSF)

Filgrastim	Sargramostim
Bone pain (usually lower back, pelvis, and sternum)	Bone pain, myalgias
Splenomegaly (in patients with chronic neutropenia)	Diarrhea, anorexia, facial flushing
Worsening of psoriasis, cutaneous vasculitis	Increased LDH, uric acid, alkaline phosphatase Rarely, thrombocytopenia

LDH = lactate dehydrogenase.

Oprelvekin (Recombinant Human Interleukin-11)

After receiving FDA approval in 1997, oprelvekin (recombinant human interleukin-11 [rh IL-11]) was made available. Oprelvekin (Neumega) is a thrombopoietic growth factor that directly stimulates the growth and proliferation of hematopoietic stem cells and megakaryocytic progenitor cells and induces megakaryocytic maturation that results in platelet production. Oprelvekin is produced in *E. coli*, its molecular mass is 19,000 D, and it is nonglycosylated. Human IL-11 is produced by bone marrow stromal cells and is part of the cytokine family that shares the gp^{130} signal transduction pathway. Two randomized, double-blind placebo-controlled studies confirmed that oprelvekin prevents severe thrombocytopenia after single or repeated doses of myelosuppressive chemotherapy regimens (3,4). When oprelvekin was studied in the setting of autologous bone marrow transplantation, it did not enhance platelet recovery. Thus, the indication for oprelvekin is the prevention of severe thrombocytopenia and reduced need for platelet transfusion after myelosuppressive chemotherapy in patients with nonmyeloid malignancies who are at high risk for severe thrombocytopenia. Oprelvekin is administered 6 to 24 hours after the completion of chemotherapy at 50 µg/kg subcutaneously. Toxicities include fluid retention, transient atrial fibrillation caused by fluid retention, blurred vision, and rashes at the injection site. Anaphylaxis or other severe adverse allergic reactions have not been reported.

Thrombopoietin

In 1994, the c-*mpl* proto-oncogene was implicated in megakaryocytic growth and differentiation; furthermore, the product of the c-*mpl* gene is the thrombopoietin receptor.

Subsequently, thrombopoietin was cloned and sequenced. Recombinant human thrombopoietin (rh-Tpo) produces an increase in megakaryocyte number, size, and ploidy, all of which contribute to increased platelet production. Thrombopoietin acts on primitive, multipotential hematopoietic progenitors. A low level of platelet production occurs in mice that lack thrombopoietin or its receptor, indicating that thrombopoietin is not necessary for platelet maturation or release into the circulation. The increase in platelet volume that occurs early in experimental thrombocytopenia may be a thrombopoietin response.

Thrombopoietin is synthesized primarily in the liver, with secondary synthesis in the kidney and in the marrow. Circulating thrombopoietin is regulated via its consumption by platelets and megakaryocytes. Currently, rh-Tpo is in clinical trials.

Transfusion Medicine

There are instances when patients with malignancies require transfusions of either erythrocytes or platelets. Because transfusions of either erythrocytes or platelets carry risks, there must be an appropriate indication for transfusion.

Platelet Transfusions

Over the past few years, there has been controversy over what platelet count necessitates a platelet transfusion. The former platelet threshold necessitating platelet transfusion was 20,000 cells/µL. The level was taken from data derived from patients with myeloid leukemia in the mid-1960s. Based on that report, patients with myeloid leukemia with a platelet count of less than 20,000 cells/µL and a leukocyte count in excess of 100,000 cells/µL had an inordinately high risk of central nervous system bleeding (5). Over the past few years, based on the observations in patients with chronic thrombocytopenia who rarely developed spontaneous bleeding even when the platelet counts were 2000 to 3000 cells/µL, there has been a re-examination of what platelet levels should prompt prophylactic platelet transfusions. Some experts have argued that a platelet count of less than 5000 cells/µL should represent the threshold (6). A recent randomized study in patients with AML and chemotherapy-induced thrombocytopenia has proved that the risk of spontaneous bleeding is no greater when the platelet count is allowed to decrease to 5000 cells/µL or less than when the threshold is 20,000 cells/µL or less (7). Therefore, it appears that platelet transfusions should be administered to patients who are otherwise stable when the platelet count reaches 5000 cells/µL or less.

This rules does not apply to patients who are thrombocytopenic (<50,000 cells/µL) and who are actively bleeding. Platelets should be transfused in such patients to achieve a platelet count of 50,000 cells/µL or greater with the aid of platelet transfusion.

Platelet transfusion can revoke febrile reactions owing to leukocytes contaminating platelet product. Additionally, in an immunocompromised and immunosuppressed patient, one can transmit cytomegalovirus (CMV) via platelet transfusions. Leukocyte filters deplete white blood cell contamination with a 99.9% efficacy and minimize the febrile reactions, allergic reactions, and transmission of CMV.

How to Order Platelets

I prefer to use platelets from single donors, if available, rather than random-donor (pooled) platelets. One unit of single-donor platelets is equivalent to 6 U of random-donor platelets. The platelets should be filtered (leukopoor) to minimize any potential reactions or transmission of CMV. For patients receiving the first transfusion it is not necessary to premedicate with steroids or diphenhydramine; however, acetaminophen, 650 mg, is advised. The efficacy of a platelet transfusion is defined by the platelet increment, platelet survival, platelet function, and clinical evaluation of hemostasis. A useful method for determining the platelet increment is drawing a 1-hour post-transfusion platelet count and determining the corrected platelet count increment (CCI) (Fig. 5-3).

For example, if a patient with a body surface area of 1.7 m^2 and a pre–platelet transfusion count of 6000 cells/µL receives a single unit of platelets containing 4.5×10^{11} cells (the number is provided by the blood bank), and has a 1-hour post-transfusion platelet count of 24,000 cells/µL, then the CCI is 24,000 minus 6000 = 18,000 divided by 4.5 multiplied by 1.7 = a CCI of 6800. By the CCI criterion, a CCI of less than 7500 at 1 hour after platelet transfusion represents an unsuccessful transfusion with only a 15% to 25% recovery rate of the transfused platelets.

A CCI of 7500 or greater at 1 hour represents a successful transfusion with a 25% to 30% recovery rate. Patients with a CCI of 7500 or less require evaluation for the causes of platelet refractoriness, as outlined in Figure 5-4.

As outlined in the algorithm, the first step would be to use platelets from an ABO-compatible donor. Because erythrocytes always contaminate platelets, ABO-incompatible erythrocytes may cause alloimmunization and may contribute to platelet refractoriness. If platelets from ABO-compatible donors do not improve the response to platelet transfusion, fresh platelets (<24-hour shelf life) should be used. If this proves unsuccessful, it is assumed that the patient is alloimmunized to HLA and antibody testing (to both platelet and lymphocyte panels) should be conducted. If the antibody testing is positive, HLA matched from either random donors or family members should be used. If an HLA-matched donor cannot be found and a patient is at risk for spontaneous bleeding (<5000 platelets/µL), then intravenous IgG, 400 mg/kg for 3 days, with platelets from an ABO-compatible donor should be used.

There are patients who have abnormal responses to transfused platelets and who are not alloimmunized (antibody test negative, see Fig. 5-4). Reasons for

$$CCI = \left(\frac{\text{1-hour post-transfusion platelet count (cells/µL)} - \text{preplatelet transfusion count}}{\text{platelet count of transfused product (expressed as } 10^{11})} \right) \times BSA$$

Figure 5-3 Corrected platelet count increment (CCI). BSA = body surface area.

nonimmune refractoriness include platelets stored for more than 36 hours, splenomegaly, fever, and acute or chronic disseminated intravascular coagulation (DIC). In these instances, the best recourse is to attempt to treat or manage the underlying defect (i.e., fever, DIC) and to use either single-donor platelets every 12 hours or random-donor platelets (4–6 U) every 6 to 8 hours.

Red Blood Cell Transfusions

In 1977, approximately 12 million units of blood were transfused in the United States. The number of units transfused since the mid-1980s has

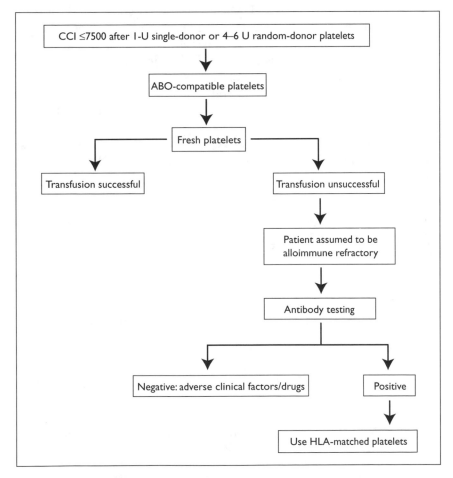

Figure 5-4 Management of platelet-refractory patients. CCI = corrected platelet count increment; HLA = human lymphocyte antigens.

leveled off. The reason is clearly related to the recognition that blood transfusions can transmit human immunodeficiency virus. The risk/benefit ratio needs to be factored in every time a unit of blood is transfused, and transfusion must be firmly indicated. In patients with cancer, the availability of human recombinant erythropoietin (discussed earlier in this chapter) has already decreased the number of units of blood transfused to patients with solid tumors. In contrast, the transfusion needs of patients with hematologic malignancies and myeloproliferative disorders remain unchanged.

Whole blood that is donated is collected in cPDA-1, an anticoagulant, and has a shelf life of 35 days. The volume of a unit of whole blood is 510 mL (450 mL of blood and 63 mL cPDA-1). Within 24 hours of collection of a unit of whole blood, the leukocytes and platelets are dysfunctional and the plasma coagulant protein levels decrease. The indications for whole blood transfusions are volume deficit and exchange transfusions (Table 5-8).

Patients with malignancies who require transfusion are given packed red blood cells (PRBCs). I use a hemoglobin of less than 8.5 g/dL or hematocrit of less than 25% as the threshold for transfusion because the cardiovascular effects of anemia rarely develop until the hematocrit is less than 25%. Patients with solid tumors and a hematocrit less than 25% are given leukocyte-depleted (leukopoor) PRBCs. Leukocytes can be depleted in a variety of ways; however, the most common method is the use of filters (i.e., PALL™). Leuko-

Table 5-8 Characteristics of and Indications for Blood Tranfusions

Component	Characteristics	Indications
Whole blood	High volume	Hemorrhage Exchange transfusions Volume deficit
Packed red blood cells	Low volume	Erythrocyte deficit
Washed red blood cells	Plasma depletion Leukocyte depletion Short shelf life (<24 h)	Prevents severe allergic reactions Prevents anaphylaxis in IgA deficiency
Frozen red blood cells	Long-term storage Plasma and leukocyte depletion Must use within 24 h of thaw	Autologous storage for postponed surgery Rare donor unit storage
Irradiated red blood cells	Destroys lymphocytes	Prevents graft-versus-host disease

cyte filters greatly diminish febrile reactions and prevent transmission of CMV. Generally, one should transfuse enough units of PRBCs to increase the hemoglobin to at least 10 g/dL (usually 2 U).

In patients with hematologic malignancies (acute myeloid leukemia, acute lymphocytic leukemia, chronic myelocytic leukemia, chronic lymphocytic leukemia, myeloma, lymphoma) or patients undergoing autologous or allogenic bone marrow transplantation, I prescribe irradiated leukopoor PRBCs. The rationale is that in these patients there is a small but very real risk of transfusion-induced graft-versus-host disease from the infused donor leukocytes. The same transfusion thresholds are used (hematocrit <25%). Patients with agnogenic myeloid metaplasia or myelodysplasia probably do not require irradiated PRBCs.

Patients with acquired immunodeficiency syndrome or patients who are pregnant should receive either leukopoor PRBCs or units from CMV-negative donors to minimize transmission of CMV.

Patients receiving chronic transfusion therapy should also receive desferrioxamine to prevent iron overload.

Transfusion Reactions

Reactions to PRBCs and platelets include the following:

1. Acute reactions. These reactions are characterized by the occurrence of *fever and hives without hemolysis.* Acute reactions are the result of antibodies to donor leukocytes. The use of leukocyte filters ameliorates the potential of this reaction. The reaction is secondary to cytokine release (e.g., interleukin-1, interleukin-6, tumor necrosis factor).

2. Hemolytic reactions. These are related to erythrocyte incompatibility and can cause mortality in 5% to 10% of patients. The symptoms are chills, fever, hemoglobinemia, hemoglobinuria, flank pain, and dyspnea and can ultimately lead to DIC, multi-organ failure, and death.

3. Urticaria reactions develop in 1% to 3% of patients receiving either PRBC or platelet transfusions. The mechanism is poorly understood but is believed to be a result of recipient antibodies to donor plasma. The manifestation is hives.

4. Transfusion-related volume overload.

5. Anaphylactic shock. This is a rare reaction to PRBCs . The mechanism is poorly understood but is thought to be related to preformed recipient anti-IgA antibodies. In many instances no cause can be detected.

Treatment of transfusion reaction consists of *stopping the transfusion immediately, infusion of normal saline [maintain blood pressure, heart rate, adequate airway], reporting the reaction to transfusion to the blood bank, checking blood and urine for hemoglobin, and performing direct antiglobulin tests (Coombs and anti-C3b).*

REFERENCES

1. **Miller JA, Beveridge RA.** A comparison of GM-CSF versus G-CSF in the therapeutic setting of chemotherapy-induced neutropenia [Abstract]. Blood 1994;84:229.
2. **Nemunaitis J, Singer JW, Buckner CD, et al.** Use of recombinant human granulocyte-macrophage colony-stimulating factor in autologous marrow transplantation for lymphoid malignancies. Blood. 1988;72:834–6.
3. **Isaacs C, Robert NJ, Bailey FA, et al.** Randomized placebo-controlled study of recombinant human interleukin-11 to prevent chemotherapy-induced thrombocytopenia in patients with breast cancer receiving dose-intensive cyclophosphamide and doxorubicin. J Clin Oncol. 1997;15:3368-77.
4. **Tepler I, Elias L, Smith JW II, et al.** A randomized placebo-controlled trial of recombinant human interleukin-11 in cancer patients with severe thrombocytopenia due to chemotherapy. Blood. 1996;87:3607-14.
5. **Higby DJ, Cohen E, Holland JF, Sinks L.** The prophylactic treatment of thrombocytopenic leukemic patients with platelets: a double blind study. Transfusion. 1974;14:440–6.
6. **Beutler E.** Platelet transfusions: the 20,000/μL trigger. Blood. 1993;81:1411.
7. **Rebulla P, Finazzi G, Marangoni F, et al.** A multicenter randomized study of the threshold for prophylactic platelet transfusions in adults with acute myeloid leukemia. Gruppo Italiano Malattie Ematologiche Maligne dell'Adulto. N Engl J Med. 1997;337:1870-5.

Chapter 6

Palliative Care

A fundamental and unshakable fear that most Americans have about cancer is that the process of dying will be painful. Over the past two decades, Americans have begun to feel that sustaining life through the use of expensive technology when quality of life cannot be restored diminishes the sanctity of life. Moreover, most Americans believe that life supported artificially through the use of these technologies is morally and ethically wrong. Prominent court cases such as that of Karen Ann Quinlan in the early 1970s and others have helped focus the attention of the American public on the "right to die" and on end-of-life issues.

The fact that a significant number of patients have "living wills" and durable power of attorney with respect to health care issues is testimony that many of us have given thought to the issue of futile care and the "right to die with dignity."

Another issue that has stirred public debate and controversy is physician-assisted suicide (PAS) and euthanasia. The ethos of medicine has long been interpreted as prohibiting physicians from any behavior that would deliberately hasten a patient's demise. During the past several decades, technologic advances in the ability to sustain life have stimulated debates among patients, doctors, clergy, and ethicists regarding the withholding of life-sustaining treatment or its withdrawal as directed by a competent patient or patient surrogate. A recent Supreme Court decision supports the physician's use of intensive drugs including narcotics to manage pain and suffering. Moreover, the Supreme Court upheld the right of states to pass PAS legislation. Currently, Oregon is the only state where PAS is legal.

The American Society of Clinical Oncology stated in a policy paper that "the most important response to the public debate over PAS is to take every possible measure to assure that all physicians are well trained in optimal end-of-life care, and that all barriers to the delivery of optimal end-of-life care be removed."

All physicians need to be knowledgeable about pain control; furthermore, there can no longer be a stigma about prescribing or using opiates to relieve pain. Physicians must look at opiates for what they are, another useful category of drug, and prescribe them in a rational manner and at optimal doses.

Pain Control

Pain is one of the most frequent symptoms of patients with malignancies. As many as 30% to 50% of patients receiving active therapy and 60% to 90% of patients with advanced disease have pain.   Pain is perceived as the most dreaded consequence of cancer by patients and physicians alike. At present, the most effective treatment, particularly in patients with cancer, is a multidisciplinary one using a wide array of medical personnel. The goal of pain therapy in a patient with cancer is to *allow the patient to function at a level that he or she chooses and to die pain free.* As in any other aspect of medicine, a covenant of trust must be established between the patient and the physician. The patient expects the physician to respect the complaint of pain, to assess its severity and cause, and to determine the optimal treatment.

Barriers to cancer pain relief still remain, and these barriers include the the physician's lack of knowledge of analgesics, lack of understanding of the pathophysiology of cancer pain, and fear of the patient's addiction to narcotics. Similarly, patients often under-report the severity of their pain or fail to communicate whether the analgesics prescribed are truly relieving the pain. Patients associate narcotic use with the stigma attached to them and will only take them when the pain episodes are severe.

The treatment of cancer pain is based on a better understanding of the pain response. The pain response is mediated by excitation of peripheral receptors of thinly myelinated A-delta fibers and unmyelinated C fibers whose respective cell bodies are in the dorsal root ganglion. Their axons enter the spinal cord via the dorsal root and either ascend or descend and ultimately synapse on specific lamina in the dorsal horn. From the point of synapse, there is an extensive branched system of afferent fibers that play a role in pain modulation. Within the dorsal horn, ascending pathways arise from second-order dorsal neurons to become the neospinothalamic and paleospinothalamic tracts that project to regions of the thalamus and cortex. The neospinothalamics help localize pain and determine intensity; the paleospinothalamics are involved in arousal and the emotional components of pain. An important inhibitory pathway originates at the periaqueductal grey nuclei of the midbrain, synapses with the raphe magnus nucleus of the medulla, and projects to the dorsal horn to modulate pain transmission. Another descending pathway that modulates pain starts at the locus ceruleus and descends to the dorsal horn. Neurotransmitters such as substance P, glutamate, aspartate, adenosine diphosphate, dopamine, serotonin, norepinephrine, and the endogenous opioids, enkephalin, β-endorphin, and dynorphin all play a role in modulating the activity along the pain pathways at the spinal and supraspinal levels. The opiate receptors of the brain bind endogenous (enkephalin, β-endorphin, dynorphin) and exogenous opioids. The subpopulation of opioid receptors include high-affinity and low-affinity receptors (μ, δ, κ, σ). These subsets of opioid receptors modulate analgesia at different levels; for example, μ-receptors modulate supraspinal analgesia, whereas δ-receptors have a predominantly spinal effect. In determining the appropriate analgesic approach, the type of pain needs to be identified (Table 6-1). Although most patients with cancer have a mix of somatic and visceral pain, as many as 15% to 20% experience neuropathic pain. Neuropathic pain does not respond to the usual measures that are used in the treatment of somatic or visceral pain.

In approaching a cancer patient with pain, the physician should

1. Believe the patient's report of pain and take a serious and sincere interest in treating it
2. Take a careful history and conduct a thorough physical examination, including a detailed neurologic examination
3. Evaluate the patient's psychologic state
4. Order the appropriate diagnostic studies (e.g., bone scan, magnetic resonance imaging, radiography, computed tomography)
5. Start treatment while the patient is undergoing the work-up
6. Reassess the response to pain therapy
7. Individualize the diagnostic and therapeutic approach

Table 6-1 Types of Pain

Somatic pain (bone, muscle, myofascial)
  Dull, achy, but well localized
Visceral pain (discomfort that is organ derived from stretching, infiltration, compression of abdominal or pelvic viscera)
  Poorly localized, deep, squeezing, pressure-like, and associated with autonomic dysfunction
Neuropathic pain (injury to the central nervous system or peripheral nervous system as a consequence of tumor compression or infiltration such as a brachial or sacral plexopathy)
  Burning or dysesthetic

Pain Management

Somatic and Visceral Pain

The principles of pain management are relatively simple, and so although some physicians still find it overwhelming to treat a patient with cancer pain, it is difficult to fathom why. If the pain is somatic and mild to moderate in nature, a non-narcotic analgesic such as acetaminophen or a nonsteroidal anti-inflammatory (NSAID) is appropriate to prescribe.

Both classes of analgesics are believed to work on peripheral receptors; in the case of NSAIDs, the presumed mechanism of analgesia is mediated by inhibition of cyclooxygenase, which in turn decreases prostaglandin synthesis. The NSAIDs must be used with H_2-blockers. However, some of the newer NSAIDs have little if any predilection to ulcerate the gastric mucosa or contain drugs (Cytotec®) that protects the gastric lining. My experience is that not all NSAIDs are equivalent in relieving mild-to-moderate somatic pain in patients with cancer. Therefore, a specific NSAID should undergo a therapeutic trial of no more than 1 week. The regimens I have found useful are ibuprofen, 400 mg orally four times daily; diflusinal, 500 mg orally every 12 hours; naproxen, 500 mg orally every 12 hours, all in conjunction with the use of an H_2-blocker. If a patient responds to low-dose ibuprofen (200 mg) with a slight improvement in pain, it would be reasonable to try either a high-dose of ibuprofen or a more potent NSAID. However, if the patient experiences little improvement in somatic pain with NSAIDs alone, other pain medications must be tried. In patients with mild-to-moderate somatic or visceral pain that is unresponsive to NSAIDs, narcotic agonists/antagonists should be used. For patients with moderate pain, a combination of acetaminophen and oxycodone (5 mg) on a fixed schedule of every 3 to 4 hours is a good starting point. Recently, sustained-release forms of oxycodone (Oxy-Contin) have been introduced and can be used on a schedule of every 12 hours or every 8 hours. Again, there should be a therapeutic trial of these narcotics either in tablet or liquid form, depending on the patient's ability to swallow, with a re-evaluation after 1 week. If medication appears to offer good analgesic relief, the narcotic should be continued, while it should be kept in mind that over time patients will develop some degree of tolerance and that doses will have to be increased. The major side effects of oxycodone are drowsiness, constipation, nausea, and vomiting. Such side effects diminish the quality of life and should be treated aggressively. It is good practice to prescribe Senokot® or Peri-Colace® with a narcotic to avoid constipation. If drowsiness develops, it is reasonable to prescribe caffeine, 300 to 600 mg daily, or methylphenidate, 5 mg orally every 8 hours, or dextroamphetamine, 2.5 to 10 mg daily, to reduce the sedative effect. Nausea and vomiting, which are mediated by the effect of narcotics on the medullary chemoreceptor trigger zone, may be treated with an antiemetic.

For patients with moderate-to-severe somatic or visceral pain, the narcotic agonists/antagonists that should be used are morphine (intravenously or orally) or fentanyl (transdermally or intravenously). Morphine and hydromorphone have short half-lives (3–4 hours and 2–3 hours, respectively) and require repeated dosing. Meperidine is not superior to either morphine or hydromorphone; in fact, when meperidine is given intramuscularly, its onset of action can be as long as 1 hour. The management of severe pain requires rapid and prompt pain relief. For the hospitalized patient, a loading dose of intravenous morphine, 5 to 10 mg, followed by a continuous intravenous infusion of 1 mg/h with titration of the dose in 0.5-mg increments every few hours, achieves pain control in most patients. There are occasional patients, particularly those who have been receiving oral narcotics, who require titration at increments greater than 0.5 mg/h. In such patients, increments of 3 to 5 mg/h may be required. *There is no ceiling dose of intravenous morphine.* On rare occasions, I have personally given patients 100 to 200 mg of morphine per hour. Once the patient is stable and pain free, the 24-hour morphine dose is converted to an equivalent dose of a long-acting oral morphine preparation or, if the patient cannot swallow, transdermal fentanyl (Table 6-2).

It is important to supplement a long-acting morphine preparation of transdermal fentanyl with a short-acting oral morphine preparation such as Roxanol®, 10 to 20 mg sublingually, and to titrate the long-acting morphine dose until there is pain control. It is not adviseable to mix a long-acting oral morphine preparation with transdermal fentanyl. I prefer to use one or the other, stick with it, and titrate the dose. In the tritration process, the total oral dose of a short-acting preparation such as Roxanol is converted to either MS Contin or transdermal fentanyl based on the following equivalencies: every 10 mg of Roxanol is equiv-

Table 6-2 Morphine Equivalency Doses*

IV 24-h Morphine Dose (mg/24 h)	Oral Equivalent/Long-acting Oral Morphine (i.e., MS Contin) (mg/24 h)	Transdermal Fentanyl Equivalent (µg/h)
10–15	30–45	25
16–30	45–90	50
31–45	90–150	75
46–60	150–180	100
61–90	180–270	159
91–120	270–360	200
121–150	360–450	250
151–180	450–540	300

*60 mg/24 h morphine IV = 180 mg/24 h MS Contin PO = 100 µg/h fentanyl treatment.

alent to 10 mg of MS Contin, which in turn is equivalent to 3 μg of transdermal fentanyl. Adjunctive therapy would include the use of NSAIDs.

Neuropathic Pain

Neuropathic pain does not respond well to opoids or NSAIDs. The initial treatment of neuropathic pain involves drugs that diminish or decrease transmission along nerve fibers, such as amitryptyline, dilantin, carbamazepine, and neurontin. I prefer to use amitryptyline, 10 to 25 mg orally three times daily; carbamazepine, 100 mg orally twice or three times daily; or neuontin, 200 to 300 mg orally twice daily, and tirtrate the dose if the patient responds. Amitryptyline may cause drowsiness; methylphenidate can be used to counteract it. Carbamazepine can cause agranulocytosis and therefore monitoring of the leukocyte count is necessary. Neurontin is relatively safe but can lead to sedation. If a patient responds to these regimens but not completely, NSAIDs can be used as an adjunct. If a patient with neuropathic pain does not respond to these aforementined drugs, then a sympathetic nerve blockade (celiac for abdominal pain, superior hypogastric for pelvic pain) is one option. Other options include transepidermal neurostimulatory TENs units, intraspinal opiods, or cordotomy.

Many patients with cancer and pain are appropriately depressed. The use of antidepressants, particularly the serotonin uptake inhibitors (fluoxetine [Prozac], paroxetine [Paxil], sertraline [Zoloft]) should be used if the depression interferes with the patient's ability to function. Despite the diagnosis of cancer, it is expected that the patient be able to get up in the morning, get dressed, help in food preparation, partake in family meals, participate in family gatherings, and so on. If this partcipation in life is not occurring, then treatment with an antidepressant is indicated.

Most recently, the diphosphonate, pamidronate (Aredia) has been shown to decrease significantly the incidence of fractures and diminish bone pain in patients with myeloma and breast cancer. In patients with prostate cancer and bone metastatses, pamidronate can diminish the severity of bone pain. This agent has become an important adjunct in pain management.

Palliative Radiotherapy

Palliative radiotherapy is an effective means of treating painful bone metastases. The local radiotherapy field encompasses the area of metastases and a surrounding margin. The fractionation schemas are short-course, 5 to 15 fractions, and a low total dose of 15 to 40.5 Gy. In some radiation therapy series, 90% of patients experienced some degree of pain relief, with 54% experiencing complete pain relief. Hemibody radiation therapy (HBI), upper half or lower half, is an approach designed to deliver wide-field radiotherapy to multiple bone metastases in a single course of treatment. The fractions are 6 Gy to the upper half or 8 Gy to the lower half. In contrast to local field radiotherapy, which take as long as 3 months to render significant pain relief, HBI usually works within 48 hours, with 73% of patients experiencing some pain relief and 19% experiencing complete pain relief. Systemic radiotherapy, strontium-89 and samarium-153 lexidronam, are systemic radionuclides that deliver radiotherapy to bone. Both of these radionuclides have been shown to palliate bone pain in patients with hormone refractory prostate cancer and bone metastases. Strontium-89 is used as a 10.8 mCi dose and samarium-153 is dosed at 1.0 mCi/kg. Since both strontium-89 and samarium-153 emit no appreciable gamma radiation, the treated patient is not a hazard to family or health care workers and outpatient treatment is possible. Patients who respond to either strontium-89 or samarium-153 usually do so in a matter of weeks, and maximum pain relief occurs within 3 to 4 weeks. Both strontium-89 and samarium-153 cause leukopenia and thrombocytopenia. The counts usually return to normal within 8 weeks of treatment.

Palliative Surgery

Internal fixation of long bone fractures should be considered even in a patient who is terminally ill, provided that life expectancy is more than 1 month. This is done simply and purely to palliate pain. Patients with vertebral metastases that are causing spinal instability, with or without neurologic compromise, and with chronic pain are candidates for palliative surgery simply to alleviate pain and restore mobility.

Malignant Effusions

If a patient has a life expectancy of more than 30 days, malignant effusions are treated with thoracostomy tube drainage and pleurodesis. (The technique of thoracentesis is discussed in Chapter 3, p 63.) Video thoracoscopy and talc insufflation is a highly effective technique but requires a general anesthetic and a short hospital stay. With the advent of a flexible thoracostomy tube, it is possible to treat patients on an ambulatory basis. After the lung has expanded and the output from the thoracostomy tube is less than 100 mL/h sterile talc, bleomycin or interleukin-2 may be instilled to promote pleurodesis.

Malignant ascites is much more difficult to manage. Clearly, abdominal paracentesis has a role in affording relief of abdominal distention and bloating; however, repeated paracentesis is not advised because of the risks of infection and of potentially worsening an already existing catabolic state by further depleting protein in the ascites fluid. In patients who have a life expectancy of greater than 6 months, LaVine shunts (abdominal cavity to the superior vena cava) are a consideration in managing malignant ascites. The potential complications include shunt occlusion and chronic disseminated intravascular coagulation (DIC). Intraperitoneal chemotherapy with either cisplatin, 5-FU, or bleomycin is occasionally effective in women with malignant ascities from ovarian cancer.

Hospice Care

The hospice movement originated in Europe and has established itself in the United States over the past decade. Hospice provides palliative care to patients with cancer and today to any patient who is terminally ill. The philosophy of hospice care is symptom management including aggressive pain-relieving measures. These measures often include using narcotics at doses that achieve pain relief even if that dose leads to the toxic effects of a narcotic overdose. Hospice provides emotional and psychological support to terminally ill patients and their families. The family support is often invaluable for family members who have a difficult time coping with the loss of a family member or loved one.

Patients appropriate for hospice care include terminally ill patients with a life expectancy of 6 months or less. Referral to hospice should be done in a timely manner because both patients and families do benefit from the psychological and emotional support. Unfortunately, the sad reality is that most hospice referral occurs within days to weeks of death and the support then provided is not what it could have been. Hospice referral should take place when life expectancy is still measured in months.

Many patients perceive that hospice referral is admitting defeat; many are fearful that the referral will serve to sever ties with their physician. These fears need to be dispelled by the physician first and foremost. Hospice care does not sever ties; most hospices will allow the patient's physician to assume and actively control hospice care. Furthermore, hospice care must be presented as yet another form of active care; however, the focus of hospice is relief of symptoms as opposed to controlling the growth or eradicating a tumor. If the physician takes the lead in presenting hospice care in this framework, any resistance the patient might feel is easily overcome.

In geographic regions that do not have hospice facilities, the physician may wish to refer a patient to a hospice outside the community. In doing so, it is clear that the physician may lose control. However, the loss of control does not mean severing ties. A weekly phone call is often enough to keep the physician-patient tie intact even when another physician is in charge. A phone call with queries such as "How are you feeling today?" and "How much pain are you in?" and queries about family convey to the patient that the physician is interested and involved.

Case 6-1

A 55-year-old nurse presented to the hospital emergency room after an automobile accident for evaluation of chest trauma. She was in mild distress and reported symptoms of sternal pain. Her blood pressure was 130/94 mm Hg; respiratory rate was 24 breaths/min; heart rate was 112 beats/min and regular; and her temperature was 99.8 °F. Physical findings were tenderness over the sternum and a 4 × 6 cm hard mass in the 5 o'clock position of the right breast. A 3-cm right axillary mass was also palpable. She reported that the mass had been present for more than a year and a half. She had been fearful that it was breast cancer and had not sought medical attention. The multichannel chemistries and complete blood count were within normal limits. Chest radiography showed clear lung fields, a 10% left pneumothorax, and an obvious sternal fracture on the lateral view with a possibility of a pathologic fracture. Computed tomography of the chest confirmed a sternal fracture with the presence of lytic bone disease involving the sternum.

She was admitted to the hospital for pain control and observation of the left pneumothorax.

She underwent a core biopsy of the right breast that showed an infiltrating ductal breast cancer, estrogen/progesterone receptor negative. A bone scan showed widespread disease.

She was started on a chemotherapy regimen of cyclophosphamide and doxorubicin (CA). The response to therapy was almost complete, with resolution of her right breast mass, and axillary nodes, an improvement of her bone scan, and osteoblastic change of the previously lytic bone disease in her sternum. She continued to receive CA for 1 year after which she received paclitaxel for an additional 8 months. All therapy was then discontinued. She did well for 1 year without chemotherapy and then developed progressive bone disease. She then started treatment with vinorelbine, 5-FU, and leucovorin for 15 months, followed by continuous infusions of 5-FU for an additional 12 months. At that time all therapy was discontinued. She remained free of disease progression for 9 months, when she developed progression in bone and liver. She was given two cycles of taxotere without response. At that time, following an intensely emotional discussion with her physician, she decided to enter hospice care.

She was cared for at home with hospice care for 5 months. During this time, her bone pain was palliated with MS Contin, 90 mg orally every 12 hours. Radiation therapy was used to palliate lytic disease at T-9.

She required admission to an inpatient hospice unit when it became impossible to care for her at home. She died peacefully 27 days later.

Chapter 7

Lymphoid Neoplasia

Acute Lymphoblastic Leukemia

Acute lymphoblastic leukemia (ALL) can arise from lymphoid progenitors of either the B-cell or T-cell lineage. In most adults (70%–75%), ALL usually has a "pre–B-cell" phenotype, CD19+, CD10+ (the common acute leukemia antigen [cALL]), but lacks cytoplasmic immunoglobulins (Ig). Adults with pre–B-cell ALL may have either normal cytogenetics or the following abnormalities: 6q–, 9p–, t(9;22), t(4;11), or are hyperdiploid (see Table 1-5, p 16). A small minority of adults with ALL have a mature B-cell phenotype and are therefore designated as having a "Burkitt leukemia," which is especially prevalent in persons infected with human immunodeficiency virus. The remaining 25% or so of adults with ALL have a T-cell phenotype. Patients with T-cell ALL usually have a translocation of the T-cell receptor gene located on chromosome 7 (see Table 1-5, p 16). Adults with T-cell ALL have a poor prognosis.

Signs and Symptoms

Most adults with ALL present with signs and symptoms of pancytopenia: easy bruisability, fatigue, fever, or infection. The physical findings may show petechiae, ecchymosis, or splenomegaly. Lymphadenopathy is rarely found. Acute lymphoblastic leukemia should be suspected in patients with pancytopenia. The diagnosis is made on bone marrow aspirate and bone core biopsy. A sample of either the marrow aspirate or core biopsy should be sent for cytogenetics.

Table 7-1 Treatment of Acute Lymphoblastic Leukemia in Adults

Induction (Weeks 1–9)	CNS Prophylactic (Weeks 5–8)	Maintenance (Weeks 10–18)	Consolidation (Weeks 19–28)	Maintenance (Weeks 29–130)
Phase 1 (Weeks 1–4)				
Vincristine 2 mg/wk IVP × 4	Methotrexate 10 mg intrathecally on Days 31, 38, 45, 52	6-Mercatopurine 60 mg/m^2/d PO	Vincristine 2 mg/wk IVP	6-Mercatopurine 60 mg/m^2/d PO
Daunorubicin 25 mg/m^2/wk IVP × 4	Cranial RT 2400 cGy	Methotrexate 20 mg/m^2/wk PO or IV	Doxorubicin 25 mg/m^2/wk IV on Weeks 20, 21, 22, 23	Methotrexate 20 mg/m^2/wk PO or IV
Prednisone 60 mg/m^2/d PO for 4 wk			Dexamethasone 10 mg/m^2 PO daily for 4 wk	
L-Asparaginase 500 U/m^2 IV on Days 1–14			Cyclophosphamide 650 mg/m^2 IV on Week 24	
Phase 2 (Weeks 5–9)				
Cyclophosphamide 650 mg/m^2 every 2 wk IV on Weeks 5, 7, 9				
Cytosine arabinoside 75 mg/d on Days 31–34, 38–41, 45–48, 52–55				

Treatment and Prognosis

Although children with ALL have an excellent prognosis, the same is not true of adults. In adults with ALL, the 5-year disease-free survival is 25% to 35%, and poor prognostic features include an elevated leukocyte count at presentation, and abnormal cytogenetics such as t(9;22) or t(4;11). The goal of antileukemia therapy is to rapidly reduce the leukemic burden to a point at which it is no longer detected by clinical microscopy. This is defined as a complete remission (CR). Although the diagnosis of CR is based on clinical microscopy, it is clear that, given the vastness of the bone marrow cavity and the limited sampling of a bone marrow aspirate, one could easily miss a single lymphoblast in a field of 400 to 500 normal bone marrow cells. If one assumes that the bone marrow contains 1000 trillion cells (1×10^{12}), then the residual leukemic burden could easily be 2 to 2.5×10^{11} cells, which is still a significant leukemic burden. Clearly additional therapy (consolidation) is necessary to further reduce the residual leukemic burden. In adults with ALL, prophylactic therapy is delivered to the central nervous system, followed by maintenance therapy for 2 years. A typical regimen is shown in Table 7-1. The median survival of adults with ALL is 24 to 36 months, with a 5-year survival of 35% to 40%.

The treatment of relapsed adult ALL is a challenge and includes allogeneic bone marrow transplantation (BMT) and autologous BMT. The median survival of relapsed adults with ALL is 12 to 18 months.

Chronic Lymphatic Leukemia

Chronic lymphatic leukemia (CLL) is a malignancy that results from the clonal expansion of mature lymphocytes. The clonal malignant lymphocytes are of the B-cell lineage in 85% to 95% of cases, with the remaining 5% to 10% of cases being of the T-cell lineage. The median age at diagnosis is 65 to 75 years.

Signs and Symptoms

Most patients are asymptomatic at the time of diagnosis or have constitutional symptoms such as fatigue, weakness, or malaise. In 20% to 25% of patients, there are no physical findings, and in 75% to 80% of patients, the physical findings include lymphadenopathy, splenomegally, and, infrequently, hepatomegally.

The diagnostic criteria for CLL are:
1. Unexplained lymphocytosis, greater than 5×10^9/L with the immunophenotype of CD19+, CD20+, CD5+.
2. Atypical lymphocytes—i.e., prolymphocytes less than 55%.
3. Bone marrow lymphocytes greater than 30%.

The differential diagnosis of chronic B-cell leukemias is shown in Table 7-2. Immunohistochemical staining helps differentiate CLL from other B-cell leukemias (see Table 7-2).

Treatment and Prognosis

As shown in Table 7-3, both the Rai and Binet staging systems are predictive for survival in patients with CLL. Patients with Rai stage III or IV and Binet stage C have a limited survival and require treatment. In contrast, patients

Table 7-2 Differential Diagnosis of Chronic B-Cell Leukemias*

	CLL	Prolymphocytic Leukemia	Hairy Cell Leukemia	Follicular Lymphoma
SMIg	+	+++	+++	+++
CD22	—	++	++	+
CD19,20	++	+++	++	++
CD24	++	+++	++	++
CD10	—	—	—	+
CD25	—	—	++	—
CD38	—	—	—	—

	Intermediate Grade Lymphoma	Splenic Lymphoma with Villous Lymphocytes	Plasma Cell Leukemia
SMIg	++	+++	—
CD22	+	++	—
CD19,20	++	++	—
CD24	++	++	—
CD10	+	—	—
CD25	—	—	—
CD38	—	—	++

+ = mild staining; ++ = moderate staining; +++ = intense staining.
*After a diagnosis of CLL is made, the cancer is staged using the Rai system or the Binet system as shown in Table 7-3.

with Rai stages 0, I, II, or Binet stages A or B should be observed and require treatment only if it is indicated. Indications include progressive anemia, progressive or painful splenomegally, progressive or bulky adenopathy, rapidly increasing lymphocytosis, autoimmune hemolytic anemia or thrombocytopenia, increasing frequency of bacterial infections, or systemic symptoms such as fever, night sweats, or weight loss. When patients with CLL require treatment, fludarabine is the drug of choice. Fludarabine results in an improvement (defined as down-staging of CLL and/or an improvement in anemia or thrombocytopenia) in 80% of patients with CLL, with 60% of patients achieving a CR (defined as a complete resolution of lymphadenopathy, splenomegaly, and hepatomegaly, and a normalization of the complete blood count [CBC]). In patients achieving a CR, the bone marrow will either be entirely normal or show the presence of nodular or focal lymphocytic infiltrates. Other treatments include chlorambucil, 2-chlorodeoxyadenosine (2-cda), and bone marrow transplantation (allogeneic or autologous). The chimeric monoclonal antibody to CD20, rituximab, is currently undergoing clinical trials.

Patients with CLL are predisposed to infections as a result of hypogammaglobulinemia. However, the routine administration of intravenous gammaglobulin is not cost effective.

Table 7-3 Rai and Binet Staging System for Chronic Lymphatic Leukemia

Clinical Characteristics	Rai Stage	Modified Rai	Binet Stage	Median Survival
Lymphocytosis in the peripheral blood and marrow	0	Low	A	>10 y
Hgb >10 g/dL, patients >100,000 /µL, and <3 nodal areas involved			A	>10 y
Lymphocytosis and enlarged nodes	I	Intermediate		6 y
Lymphocytosis and enlarged spleen or liver	II	Intermediate		6 y
Hgb >10 g/dL, platelets >100,000/µL, and >3 nodal areas involved			B	6 y
Lymphocytosis and anemia Hgb <10 g/dL	III	High		2 y
Lymphocytosis and thrombocytopenia <100,000 cells/µL	IV	High		2 y
Hgb <10 g/dL, platelets <100,000/µL or both			C	2 y

Hodgkin Disease

The cause of Hodgkin disease (HD) is unknown. The transformed cell, the Reed-Sternberg cell (Fig. 7-1), is believed to be a transformed B cell of germinal center origin, and the cellular infiltrate surrounding the Reed-Sternberg cell is believed to be the "host's" immunologic response.

Hodgkin disease has two peaks in incidence, the first occurring in the second decade of life and the second occurring in the fifth decade of life.

Signs and Symptoms

The presenting symptoms are fever, night sweats, weight loss, cough, and enlarged lymph nodes. The physical findings include lymphadenopathy and mediastinal masses. The diagnosis of HD is determined by the results of a lymph node biopsy. After HD has been diagnosed, patients are clinically and pathologically staged (see Chapter 3). In addition to chest radiography, computed tomography of the chest, abdomen, and pelvis, bone marrow aspirate, and bone core biopsy, some patients may require lymphangiography and or positron emission tomography. For example, lymphangiog-

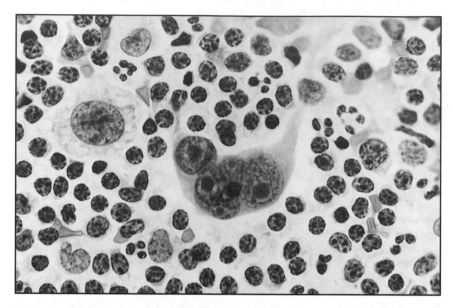

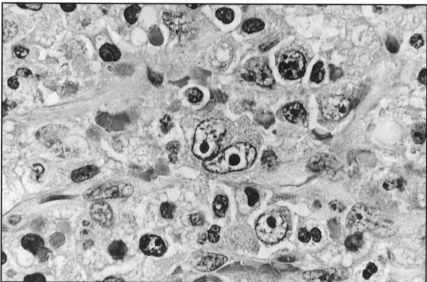

Figure 7-1 Biopsy of a lymph node showing a typical Reed-Sternberg cell on a touch preparation (*top*) and a hematoxylin and eosin section (*bottom*) (×400).

raphy is indicated in patients with lymphocyte-predominant HD who have involvement of the right cervical region (CSIA/IIA) or in patients with nodular sclerosis who have a small mediastinal mass. After staging has been completed, patients with HD are assigned a clinical/pathologic stage as shown in Table 7-4. Currently, a staging laparotomy has little if any role in the staging of HD and is no longer recommended.

Treatment and Prognosis

The treatment of HD is a function of the histologic subtype (Table 7-5), the clinical/pathologic stage, the presence or absence of symptoms (weight loss, night sweats, fever are designated as "B" symptoms), and the presence or absence of bulky mediastinal adenopathy. The treatment of HD consists of either subtotal lymphoid irradiation or chemotherapy. Chemotherapy with alkylating agents is not recommended, because it predisposes patients with HD to treatment-related leukemias. Patients with HD who can be exclusively treated with subtotal lymphoid irradiation include the following:

1. Patients with CSIA lymphocyte-predominant HD and a supradiaphragmatic presentation, usually right cervical.
2. Female patients with supradiaphragmatic CSIA or CSIIA HD and mediastinal masses whose transverse diameter is less than one third the diameter of the thorax at its widest point on a standing posteroanterior chest radiograph.
3. Patients with subdiaphragmatic CSIA HD with groin/inguinal presentations. Such presentation are extremely rare, accounting for only 2% to 3% of all patients with HD. These patients do not require staging laparotomy and can be treated with an inverted Y radiation therapy field coupled with splenic irradiation.

All other patients, CSIB, CSIIB, CSIIIA and B, PSIVA and B, and CSIIA with bulky mediastinal masses (defined as a transverse diameter that is more than one third the widest diameter of the thorax on a standing posteroanterior chest radiograph) are treated with chemotherapy.

The chemotherapy of choice is ABVD (doxorubicin 25 mg/m^2, bleomycin 10 U/m^2, vinblastine 6 mg/m^2, DTIC 375 mg/m^2, all given intravenously on

Table 7-4 Staging of Lymphoma (Hodgkin and Non-Hodgkin)

Stage		
	I	Tumor confined to a single lymph node or a single contiguous lymph node chain above or below the diaphragm
	II	Tumor confined to two contiguous lymph nodes or nodal chains above or below the diaphragm
	III	Tumor involving lymph node chains above and below the diaphragm
	IV	Involvement of parenchymal organs, such as bone marrow, liver, pleural space, or multiple sites such as skin, lung, bone, etc.
Modifiers		A - absence of fever, night sweats, weight loss >10% body weight
		B - presence of fever, night sweats, weight loss >10% body weight
		E - extranodal involvement of a single site in skin, thyroid, bone, gastrointestinal tract

Table 7-5 Histologic Subtypes of Hodgkin Disease

Lymphocyte predominant
Nodular sclerosis
Mixed cellularity
Lymphocyte depleted

Days 1 and 15 with an every-28-day treatment cycle). In patients treated with cyclic chemotherapy such as ABVD, the number of treatment cycles (every 28 days = 1 cycle) required is flexible because the end point is a CR (complete disappearance of all clinical evidence of disease). Usually this takes a minimum of six cycles. Two additional cycles are administered after a patient achieves a CR. Close to 90% of patients treated with the ABVD regimen achieve a CR, and 61% are alive without disease at 5 years. Unlike its predecessor, the MOPP (mechlorethamine [nitrogen mustard], Oncovin [vincristine], procarbazine, prednisone) regimen, the ABVD program has not been associated with treatment-induced leukemias, and the infertility/sterility rate associated with this regimen is 15% to 25%.

Long-Term Complications of Therapy

The emphasis today in treating patients with HD is to attempt to diminish the long-term complications of therapy. These include myelodysplasia and acute leukemia from MOPP chemotherapy alone or from MOPP chemotherapy used in conjunction with radiotherapy. These treatment-induced acute leukemias are associated with a chromosomal translocation between chromosomes 5 and 7 (see Chapter 1). The other long-term complications are radiation-induced malignancies: breast, lung, gastric, and thyroid cancers; melanoma; and soft tissue sarcomas. These radiation-induced malignancies typically occur 15 to 20 years after radiation therapy. Women who have received mediastinal irradiation are at risk for breast cancer, particularly bilateral breast cancer. The management of radiation-induced breast cancer or any of the radiation-induced malignancies just mentioned is identical to that of patients in whom these malignancies develop "de novo." At present, these radiation-induced second malignancies cannot be prevented; physicians need to be cognizant that long-term survivors of HD are at risk for these long-term complications of therapy.

Patients with HD who relapse after radiation therapy can be salvaged with the ABVD regimen of chemotherapy. Patients who relapse within 12 months of ABVD can be salvaged with high-dose chemotherapy and hematopoietic progenitor cell support (autologous bone marrow transplantation [ABMT]). Years after receiving the ABVD regimen, patients can be salvaged by using the MOPP regimen or vice versa (ABVD if the initial regimen was MOPP).

The two patients described in Cases 7-1 and 7-2 exemplify the diagnostic dilemmas that one encounters in the treatment of patients with HD.

Case 7-1

A 26-year-old black woman presented to her physician in 1987 with complaints of fever, night sweats, and a 3-kg weight loss over a 3-month period. The past medical history was significant for two uncomplicated pregnancies and one miscarriage. The physical findings were as follows: appearance (e.g., thin) of chronic illness; height of 152 cm: weight of 40 kg: temperature of 38.5 °C; blood pressure of 124/84 mm Hg, respiratory rate of 18 breaths/min. The pertinent findings were confined to the lymph nodal examination and revealed a left inguinal nodal mass that was 3 × 5 cm, an enlarged right inguinal node that measured 2 × 3 cm, and a right femoral node that measured 2 × 2 cm. The remainder of the lymph node examination and physical examination was unremarkable.

A biopsy of the right inguinal node helped yield a diagnosis of HD, mixed cellularity.

The following sequential staging studies were done: chest radiography, computed tomography (CT) of the chest, bone marrow examination. An abdominal/pelvic CT showed the presence of para-aortic and left iliac adenopathy. A gallium-67 scan showed increased uptake in the right and left inguinal regions, para-aortic region, and right and left iliac regions, and a normal distribution everywhere else. On the basis of these staging procedures, the patient was considered to have clinical stage IIB HD and started on MOPP chemotherapy. On completion of the six cycles of the MOPP regimen, she achieved a clinical CR; two more courses of MOPP were administered, after which all treatment ceased.

She was followed on a routine basis every 3 months. On routine surveillance chest radiography performed at the 18-month follow-up visit, asymptomatic symmetrical bilateral hilar adenopathy was detected. The results of a CBC and multichannel chemistries at the time of her visit were normal. The erythrocyte sedimentation rate was elevated at 50 mm/h. Computed tomography of the chest confirmed the presence of right and left hilar adenopathy and showed 1.5-cm nodes in the right and left paratracheal regions. The findings on abdominal and pelvic CT were normal. A gallium-67 scan showed uptake in the mediastinum, bilateral hilum, and diffuse uptake in both lungs suggestive of an inflammatory process. The serum angiotensin-converting enzyme (ACE) level was elevated.

Based on the elevated ACE level and the appearance of the gallium scan, a presumptive diagnosis of sarcoidosis was made, which was confirmed by medi-

Continued.

Case 7-1—cont'd

astinoscopy and biopsy of the right paratracheal lymph nodes (noncaseating granulomas).

The patient was treated and observed, and over a period of 12 months the bilateral hilar adenopathy spontaneously regressed.

Discussion
This patient's clinical course illustrates the two important aspects in the care of a patient with a malignancy. The first is the need to step back and restage the patient at the time of presumed relapse. The second is the need to confirm histologically a presumed relapse whenever possible. The symmetrical bilateral hilar involvement without an obvious mediastinal mass seen in this patient would be an unusual pattern of relapse in a patient with HD. Second, the gallium scan has a pattern of uptake more suggestive of an inflammatory process such as sarcoidosis. The elevated serum ACE level is suggestive of sarcoidosis but clearly not diagnostic of it. A mediastinoscopy led to the appropriate diagnosis and spared this young woman additional chemotherapy.

Case 7-2

In 1992, a 37-year-old white man presented to his internist with fatigue, occasional cough, and decreased exercise tolerance. He was an avid runner and noted over a period of a month that he was unable to perform an early morning 3-mile run without coming home feeling exhausted. He had an unproductive cough, denied hemoptysis, fever, headaches, or sweats. At the time of the physical examination, he appeared to be a well-developed, thin man in no acute distress. The pertinent physical findings included the presence of bilateral anterior and posterior cervical lymph nodes, bilateral supraclavicular adenopathy, the absence of an enlarged spleen, and the absence of any other adenopathy. The remainder of the physical examination was unremarkable.

The chest radiograph was remarkable for a large mediastinal mass. A lymph node biopsy of a right anterior cervical node helped yield a diagnosis of HD, nodular sclerosis (Fig. 7-2). Computed tomography of the chest showed the presence of a large mediastinal mass measuring 13 × 10 cm. The findings of the abdominal and pelvic CT were normal. The results of bilateral bone marrow aspirates and bone core biopsies were normal.

Based on the sequential staging studies, the patient was considered to have CSIIA HD and was started on chemotherapy with ABVD. He responded well to ABVD and attained a clinical CR. At the conclusion of six cycles of ABVD, a complete restaging once again confirmed a CR and he received two additional courses of ABVD. At the completion of the ABVD program, the patient was followed every 3

Case 7-2—cont'd

months. He did well for 18 months, at which time he developed signs and symptoms of superior vena cava syndrome. The physical findings revealed the presence of conjunctival insufflation, distension of the neck, and numerous distended veins over the upper chest, but no other abnormal physical findings. The findings of the abdominal and pelvic CT were normal. Computed tomography of the chest showed a massive mediastinal mass 18 × 15 cm and tiny nodules scattered throughout both lungs. The results of repeat bilateral bone marrow examinations were normal. A left paramediastinotomy was performed and revealed initially what was believed to be recurrent HD but on further review showed a diffuse large cell lymphoma (Fig. 7-3).

The patient was started on DHAP (dexamethasone, cytosine arabinoside, and cisplatin) chemotherapy for three cycles and attained a partial response. He then subsequently underwent ABMT, after which he achieved a CR. He has been in continuous CR for the past 50 months.

Discussion

Non-Hodgkin lymphoma is a rare second malignancy that can complicate the course of HD. In this man's situation, the occurrence of superior vena cava syndrome, which is a rare manifestation of HD, prompted the question of "Could the mediastinal mass be anything else?" That question led to the mediastinotomy and an accurate tissue diagnosis of an aplastic large cell lymphoma, B-cell subtype, with vascular invasion (angiotrophic lymphoma).

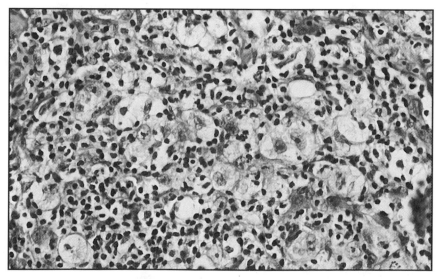

Figure 7-2 Biopsy of a right supracavicular lymph node showing Hodgkin disease, nodular sclerosis.

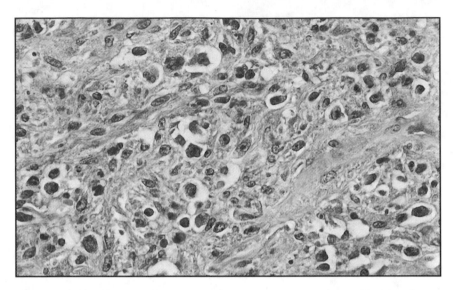

Figure 7-3 Biopsy of a mediastinal mass in a patient with previous Hodgkin disease (see Fig. 7-2), now showing malignant lymphoma, diffuse, large cell, anaplastic.

Non-Hodgkin Lymphomas

The non-Hodgkin lymphomas (NHL) represent one of the cancers that is steadily increasing in incidence. The incidence of NHL has risen from 5.9 cases per 100,000 persons in 1950 to 13.7 cases per 100,000 persons in 1999. Much of the increase in incidence is related to human immunodeficiency virus (HIV) infection and HIV-related lymphomas; however, even if one excludes the HIV-related lymphomas, the number of persons diagnosed with NHL has nonetheless increased. The incidence of NHL is slightly more prevalent in men than in women, and 23,800 deaths will occur from NHL in 2000.

The NHLs (Tables 7-6 to 7-8) represent a heterogeneous group of diseases that can arise in lymphoid tissue (lymph nodes, spleen), bone marrow, or almost any other tissue. In fact, extranodal involvement occurs in 26% of patients with NHL, and the most frequent extranodal sites are the stomach, skin, oral cavity, pharynx, small intestine, and the central nervous system. Certain subtypes of NHL appear to be endemic in specific parts of the world. In Japan and the Caribbean, for instance, human T-cell lymphoma virus (HTLV)-1–associated lymphomas appear to be prevalent (Table 7-7). Burkitt lymphoma (Working Formulation J) is endemic to Nigeria and Tanzania. In the Middle East, alpha heavy-chain disease, a lymphoma with a predilection for gastrointestinal involvement, is prevalent. Furthermore, alpha-heavy chain

Table 7-6 Working Formulation Classification for Non-Hodgkin Lymphoma

Low Grade
  A. Malignant lymphoma, diffuse, small lymphocytic
  B. Malignant lymphoma, follicular, small cleaved cell
  C. Malignant lymphoma, follicular, mixed, small and large cell

Intermediate Grade
  D. Malignant lymphoma, follicular, large cell
  E. Malignant lymphoma, diffuse, small cleaved cell
  F. Malignant lymphoma, diffuse, mixed, small and large cell
  G. Malignant lymphoma, diffuse, large cell

High Grade
  H. Malignant lymphoma, large cell, immunoblastic
  I. Malignant lymphoma, lymphoblastic
  J. Malignant lymphoma, small noncleaved cell

Table 7-7 Malignant Lymphomas Misrepresented or not Represented in the Working Formulation

Mantle cell lymphomas—misrepresented as low grade, behave as intermediate-to-high grade
Monocytoid B-cell lymphomas
T-cell lymphomas
HTLV-associated leukemia/lymphoma

disease is almost never encountered in persons other than those of Mediterranean descent. Follicular lymphomas (Working Formulation B–D) are common in the United States and Europe but are rare in the Caribbean, Africa, China, Japan, and the Middle East.

Although the cause of NHL is unknown, cytogenetic abnormalities and oncogene overexpression both play a significant role in the pathogenesis of NHL (see Chapter 1, p 9) (Table 7-9). In follicular lymphoma, the most common chromosomal abnormality is a translocation of part of the long arm of chromosome 14 (band q32, the heavy chain immunoglobulin gene locus) to chromosome 18 (at band q21). This translocation leads to the overexpression of the bcl-2 oncogene, which in turn immortalizes the cell so that programmed cell death does not occur.

Symptoms and Signs

Patients with NHL may present with a variety of symptoms, including malaise and fatigue, fever, sweats, cough, abdominal pain, or the painless enlargement of peripheral lymph nodes. In most patients, the physical findings are the presence of lymphadenopathy (see Chapter 2, p 24); however,

Table 7-8 Revised European-American Classification of Lymphoid Neoplasms (R.E.A.L. Classification)

Precursor B-cell neoplasm	Precursor T-cell neoplasm
Precursor B-lymphoblastic leukemia/ lymphoma	Precursor T-lymphoblastic lymphoma/ leukemia

Mature (peripheral) B-cell neoplasms	Mature (peripheral) T-cell neoplasms
B-cell chronic lymphocytic leukemia/small lymphocytic lymphoma	T-cell prolymphocytic leukemia
B-cell prolymphocytic leukemia	T-cell granular lymphocytic leukemia
Lymphoplasmacytic lymphoma	Aggressive NK-cell leukemia
Splenic marginal zone B-cell lymphoma	Adult T-cell lymphoma (HTLV-1+)
Hairy cell leukemia	Extranodal NK/T-cell lymphoma, nasal type
Plasma cell myeloma	Enteropathy-type T-cell lymphoma
Extranodal marginal zone B-cell lymphoma	Hepatosplenic $-\gamma\delta$ T-cell lymphoma
Mantle cell lymphoma	Subcutaneous panniculitis-like T-cell lymphoma
Follicular lymphoma	Mycosis fungoides/Sézary syndrome
Nodal marginal zone B-cell lymphoma	Anaplastic large-cell lymphoma, primary cutaneous type
Diffuse large B-cell lymphoma	Peripheral T-cell lymphoma, unspecified
Burkitt lymphoma	Angioimmunoblastic T-cell lymphoma
	Anaplastic large-cell lymphoma, primary systemic type

NK cell = natural killer cell.

Table 7-9 Chromosomal Abnormalities Associated with Non-Hodgkin Lymphoma

Neoplasm	Genes	Chromosomal Abnormalities
Non-Hodgkin		
	Igκ/*myc*	t(2;8)
	/IgH	t(2;14)
	myc/IgH	t(8;14)
	IgH/*bcl*-2	t(14;18)
B cell	IgH/*bcl*-3	t(14;19)
Mantle zone		t(14;11 q13)
MALT	IgH/*bcl*-10	t(11;14)
T cell	Tcrβ/TAL2	t(7;19)
	Tcrβ/TAN	t(7;9)
	Tcrβ/	t(7;11)
	Tcrβ/*LYL*1	t(7;19)

MALT = mucosa-associated lymphoid tissue.

some patients with NHL present with mediastinal masses and a dearth of peripheral lymphadenopathy. A minority of patients have isolated splenic enlargement or abdominal masses. The presentations of various subsets of patients with NHL are shown in Table 7-10.

Table 7-10 Common Presenting Symptoms and Signs of Patients with Non-Hodgkin Lymphoma

Non-Hodgkin Lymphoma Working Formulation Classification	Symptoms and Signs
A–C	Painless and slowly progressive lymphadenopathy. Fever, sweats, and weight loss uncommon
D–H	Peripheral lymphadenopathy; however, as many as one third have extradnodal involvement (gastrointestinal tract, skin, thyroid, central nervous system, bone marrow) "B" symptoms in 30%–40%
G	As many as 25% of patients may present with mediastinal masses and SVC syndrome
I	Mediastinal masses, SVC syndrome, cranial nerve palsy caused by leptomeningeal involvement
J	Large abdominal masses or bowel obstruction

SVC = superior vena cava.

Table 7-11 Sequential Staging Work-up for Lymphoma

Radiography
Computed tomography
Chest
Abdomen
Pelvis
Positron emission tomography (possible)
Bone marrow aspirate + core biopsies

The diagnosis of NHL relies on excisional lymph node biopsy (see Chapter 3, p 45), biopsy of a mediastinal mass, or an extranodal site. After a histologic diagnosis has been obtained, the patient is clinically staged (see Table 7-4), and sequential staging procedures are carried out (Table 7-11). In addition to these sequential staging procedures, molecular and cytogenetic analyses should be performed on the excised lymph node or bone marrow, because these studies may yield important prognostic information.

Treatment and Prognosis

Treatment of Low-Grade Lymphomas

Initial therapy of patients with NHL varies and is based on the pathologic findings. In patients with low-grade lymphoma (Working Formulation A–C), an initial period of *watching and waiting* may be appropriate; however, watching and waiting is not an option for patients with retroperitoneal masses and obstructive uropathy or for patients with hemolytic anemia, thrombocytopenia, or leukopenia. As many as 30% of patients with low-grade lymphoma may experience a spontaneous regression of their lymphoma. Indications for therapy include the presence of painful bulky lymphadenopathy, hemolytic anemia, splenomegally, or a cytopenia. In such cases, the purpose of therapy is palliation of symptoms. Cure of patients with low-grade NHL is not a reality at this time. Effective treatment includes local radiation therapy to bulky lymphadenopathy, or single-agent fludarabine, mitoxantrone, or chlorambucil. Rituximab, a chimeric murine monoclonal antibody directed against the CD-20 epitope expressed on normal "B" lymphocytes and almost all of the neoplastic lymphocytes in patients with low-grade NHL, has recently been approved by the FDA. When rituximab binds with the CD-20 epitope, it triggers apoptosis, or programmed cell death. The current indication for rituximab is low-grade NHL in patients who experience a relapse after chemotherapy. Rituximab is highly effective in these patients, and it is clear that in the future it will become first-line therapy. The toxicities of rituximab include potential allergic reactions such as anaphylaxis, hives, hypotension, and fever. Severe allergic reactions preclude continued use; however, even moderate reactions such as fever and hypotension are "first-dose" phenomena and resolve with continued therapy. The median survival for all patients with low-grade NHL is 7 to 10 years.

Treatment of Intermediate-Grade Lymphomas

All of the intermediate-grade lymphomas require immediate therapy, because without treatment the median survival is quite limited—6 to 9 months. This subset of NHL is potentially curable, and a cure is the foremost objective. The treatment of intermediate-grade NHL involves the use of multi-drug chemotherapy. The stage of intermediate-grade NHL helps determine which patients may additionally receive radiation therapy. Approximately 16% of all patients with intermediate-grade NHL are found to have CSI or CSII disease based on sequential staging studies. These patients should be treated with a brief course of multi-drug chemotherapy, which includes cyclophosphamide, doxorubicin, vincristine, and prednisone (CHOP) for four to six courses, followed by radiation therapy that encompasses all areas of involved disease. The 5-year disease-free survival rate in patients with CSI or II intermediate-grade NHL is 78% to 95%.

Patients with CSIII or CS/PS IV intermediate-grade NHL are best treated with the CHOP regimen. The CHOP regimen is as good as other multi-drug regimens that have a greater potential for toxicities. The use of CHOP in this patient group is associated with a CR rate of 65% and a 10-year disease-free survival rate of 45%. Although CHOP is standard therapy for patients with CSIII or CS/PS IV intermediate-grade NHL, more than one third fail to achieve a CR and less than 50% have a curative outcome. For patients who fail to achieve a CR or who experience a relapse after CHOP and do not have HIV-related lymphomas, a salvage regimen such as DHAP or mitoxantrone, ifosfamide, mesna, and etoposide (MIME) should be employed. In patients who are otherwise healthy, high-dose chemotherapy with autologous bone marrow transplantation (ABMT) should be administered after the use of a salvage regimen, provided that the patient responds to the salvage program. The use of ABMT in patients with relapsed intermediate-grade NHL is associated with a 5-year disease-free survival of 55% to 65%. Figure 7-4 shows the potential outcomes of patients with intermediate-grade NHL who are younger than 60 years of age.

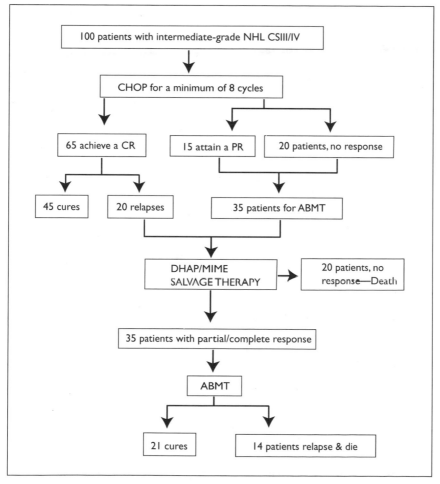

Figure 7-4 Outcomes of 100 patients with intermediate-grade non-Hodgkin lymphoma. NHL = non-Hodgkin lymphoma; CHOP = cyclophosphamide, doxorubicin, vincristine, and prednisone; CR = complete response; PR = partial response; ABMT = autologous bone marrow transplantation; DHAP = dexamethasone, cytosine arabinoside, and cisplatin; MIME =mitoxantrone, ifosfamide, mesna, and etoposide.

Treatment of High-Grade Lymphomas

Malignant lymphoma, diffuse small noncleaved are the fastest growing and most aggressive of all cancers. Patients with high-grade NHL require intensive and aggressive therapy with a CHOP-like program that includes high-dose methotrexate with leucovorin (tetrahydrofolic acid) rescue and intrathecal methotrexate, because the risk of central nervous system relapse is high. The Stanford Protocol is shown in Table 7-12. Similarly, patients with lymphoblastic lymphoma require aggressive therapy (Table 7-13) similar to that used in patients with ALL.

Patients with high-grade NHL and high-risk features (elevated serum LDH level, bone marrow involvement, or large tumor masses [>10 cm]) require autologous or allogeneic BMT while in first complete response or if only a partial response to therapy is achieved.

Special Considerations

The treatment recommendations that have been discussed in this section are specifically aimed for patients younger than 65 years old with intermediate-grade NHL who have a good performance status and are at low or intermediate risk for relapse. Patients at high risk for relapse (those with a high serum lactate dehydrogenase [LDH] level or those who are not fully ambulatory [i.e., have a performance status <70%]) should be offered participation in clinical trials that offer dose intensive therapies.

Elderly patients (>65 years) should have a thorough evaluation of cardiac, pulmonary, and renal function before the initiation of therapy. In the event that cardiac or pulmonary function is compromised, an alternative is a nonanthracycline–containing regimen such as cyclophosphamide, vincristine, procarbazine, and prednisone (COPP), or substituting mitoxantrone for doxorubicin in the CHOP program (CNOP), or using a cardioprotectant such as Zinecard with the CHOP regimen. Bleomycin is contraindicated in patients with compromised pulmonary function.

Table 7-12 Stanford Protocol for Small Noncleaved Lymphomas

Cyclophosphamide	1200 mg/m² IV Day 1 every 21 days
Vincristine	1.4 mg/m² IV Day 1 every 21 days
Doxorubicin	40 mg/m² IV Day 1 every 21 days
Prednisone	40 mg/m² PO Days 1–5 every 21 days
Allopurinol	300 mg PO Days 1-10 for 10 days
Methotrexate	3000 mg/m² IV Day 10 after 21 days
Leucovorin	25 mg/m² PO q6h for 12 doses 24 hours after methotrexate
Methotrexate	**Cycles 2 and 4**: 12 mg intrathecally Days 1 and 10

Treatment cycle = 21 days.

Table 7-13 Treatment Protocol for Lymphoblastic Lymphoma

Cyclophosphamide	400 mg/m^2 PO Days 1–3 of Weeks 1, 4, 9, 12, 15, 18
Doxorubicin	50 mg/m^2 IV Weeks 1, 4, 9, 12, 15, 18
Vincristine	1.4 mg/m^2 IV Weeks 1, 4, 9, 12, 15, 18
Prednisone	40 mg/m^2/d PO for 4 weeks, taper off on Weeks 5 and 6, then PO for 5 d Weeks 9, 12, 15, 18
Cotrimoxazole	2 tablets/d PO for 21 weeks
L-Asparaginase	6000 U/m^2 IM for 5 doses Weeks 3 and 4
Methotrexate	12 mg intrathecally Week 3, then twice weekly on Weeks 5 and 6, once on Week 7
	30 mg/m^2/d PO Weeks 21–52
6-Mercatopurine	75 mg/m^2/d PO Weeks 21–52

Patients with HIV-related lymphomas usually have intermediate-grade NHL. Rarely do patients with HIV-related lymphomas have low-grade NHL; however, if a patient with a low-grade HIV-related lymphoma is encountered, the treatment approach is exactly the same as for patients with non-HIV–related low-grade NHL. The treatment approach to patients with intermediate-grade HIV-related lymphomas is similar to that of patients with intermediate-grade NHL, namely the use of a multi-drug chemotherapy such as CHOP; however, the doses used are generally lower owing to the poor bone marrow tolerance that results from the HIV infection and the antiviral drugs used to treat it. Generally, the chemotherapy doses are about 33% lower. There are ongoing National Cancer Institute clinical trials attempting to determine the best therapy for patients with HIV-related lymphomas, and such patients should be encouraged to participate in these studies.

Patients with mantle cell lymphomas by definition fall into the low-grade category according to the Working Formulation. However, mantle cell lymphomas are biologically aggressive. Patients with mantle cell lymphomas treated with the CHOP regimen rarely achieve long-lived complete remissions (complete response). Prognostic factors associated with a limited survival in patients with mantle cell lymphomas are age greater than 60 years, diffuse histologic features, elevated serum LDH level, and peripheral blood involvement. Patients younger than 65 years with mantle cell lymphomas should be treated with CHOP to complete response or to best partial response followed by autologous or allogeneic BMT.

Multiple Myeloma

Multiple myeloma is a malignant clonal proliferation of plasma cells; plasma cells are the most differentiated forms of the lymphocyte lineage. In 2000, the

estimate is that 13,800 new cases of myeloma will be diagnosed and an estimated 10,900 Americans will die of myeloma. Multiple myeloma is a disease
of the elderly. The median age at diagnosis is 60 to 65 years, with a male predominance. The cause of multiple myeloma is unknown; however, a few
groups have found the presence of herpes virus 8 in the bone marrow dendritic cells of patients with multiple myeloma. The bone marrow dendritic
cells infected by herpes virus 8 produce interleukin-6, which is a cytokine that
serves as a plasma cell growth factor.

Although herpes virus 8 does not cause the malignant transformation of
plasma cells, it may play an important role in promoting myeloma. Patients
with monoclonal gammopathy of unknown significance (MGUS) are at risk
(1.5% per year) on a cumulative basis to develop myeloma, Waldenström
macroglobulinemia, or amyloidosis.

Symptoms and Signs

The clinical features of multiple myeloma are typically bone pain (spontaneous fractures of the ribs or vertebral bodies), anemia, hypercalcemia (nausea, fatigue, confusion, polyuria, constipation), renal failure, or recurrent
infections (usually *Streptococcus pneumoniae, Staphylococcus aureus, Haemophilus influenza*). A minority of patients are asymptomatic at the time of diagnosis. The
diagnosis is based on laboratory abnormalities. The physical findings may include pallor, localized back tenderness, or a completely normal physical examination.

The work-up for a patient in whom multiple myeloma or MGUS is suspected includes: a CBC, multichannel chemistries (blood urea nitrogen, creati-
nine, calcium), serum protein electrophoresis with quantitative immunoglobulin
levels, 24-hour urine protein and protein electrophoresis, bone marrow aspirate, and radiographic skeletal survey. The diagnosis of multiple myeloma relies on the bone marrow aspirate, which typically shows an increase in plasma
cells (>15%). The plasma cells are positive for CD38, a plasma cell antigen,
and cytoplasmic immunoglobulin (cIg). The monoclonal protein may be an
IgG (60%), IgA (20%), IgD (2%), IgE (<0.1%), and light chain κ or λ only
(18%). Biclonal elevations of myeloma proteins occur in fewer than 1% of patients and fewer than 5% of patients have nonsecretory disease.

Treatment and Prognosis

After a diagnosis of multiple myeloma is made, patients are staged based on
the Durie-Salmon staging system (Table 7-14), which attempts to define the
stage or the myeloma cell mass on the degree of anemia, the quantity of paraprotein produced, the presence or absence of hypercalcemia, and the extent of

Table 7-14 Durie-Salmon Staging System for Myeloma

Stage	Criteria	Myeloma Cell Mass
I	Hemoglobin >10 g/dL Serum Ca: normal Normal bone radiographs or solitary lytic lesion IgG <5000 mg/dL, IgA <3000 mg/dL Bence Jones protein <4000 mg/24h	Low
II	Hemoglobin <10 g >8.5 g/dL Osteopenic bone or few lytic lesions on radiographs IgG >5000 mg <7000 mg/dL, IgA >3000 mg <5000 mg/dL	Intermediate
III	Hemoglobin <8.5 g/dL Serum calcium >12 mEq/L Multiple lytic bone lesions IgG >7000 mg/dL, IgA >5000 mg/dL Bence Jones protein >12 g/24h	High

bone disease. Other prognostic variables include the serum LDH, beta-2 microglobulin level, and chromosomal abnormalities. The stage of myeloma influences which therapy is ultimately chosen.

Treatment and Response Criteria

For symptomatic patients with stage I myeloma, melphalan and prednisone (M&P) on an intermittent basis is treatment enough. Asymptomatic patients with stage I myeloma do not need to be treated until symptoms develop. The melphalan dose is 8 mg/m^2/d orally for 4 days with prednisone 100 mg orally for 4 days. For patients with stage II or III myeloma or for any patient with myeloma and renal failure regardless of stage, the treatment is multi-drug chemotherapy with vincristine, 0.4 mg continuous IV over a 24-hour period for 96 hours; doxorubicin, 9 mg/m^2 continuous IV over a 24-hour period for 96 hours; and dexamethasone, 40 mg/d orally on Days 1 through 4, 9 through 12, and 17 through 20 (VAD). Patients receiving the VAD regimen should also receive pamidronate 90 mg IVPB monthly. Response to melphalan and prednisone or VAD is defined based on the response criteria shown in Table 7-15.

For patients with stage I myeloma who respond to therapy with M&P, treatment is usually continued for 12 to 18 months and then stopped. Melphalan and prednisone can be resumed when the paraprotein and/or symptoms of the myeloma re-emerge. The median survival for all patients with stage I myeloma is 36 months. For patients with a response to M&P, the median survival is 60 months. The median survival for all patients with stage II and III myeloma ranges from 7 to 50 months, depending on response to VAD chemotherapy. The median survival is 32 to 50 months for patients who respond to VAD and

Table 7-15 Response Criteria to Chemotherapy in Myeloma

Partial Response	>75% reduction in myeloma protein
	>95% reduction in Bence Jones protein
	<5% bone marrow plasma cells
Complete Response	All of the above plus the disappearance of serum M protein and Bence Jones protein by immunofixation
	No plasma cells in bone marrow

only 7 to 17 months for patients who do not respond to VAD. Patients of any age with stage II or III myeloma are candidates for clinical trials of autologous BMT, and patients younger than 55 years of age are candidates for clinical trials of allogeneic BMT. Phase II (feasibility) studies of ABMT in patients with stage II myeloma appear promising, and one large European randomized study in patients with stage II and III myeloma has already demonstrated the superiority of ABMT over continuous chemotherapy.

Patients with unresponsive disease can benefit from treatment with high-dose dexamethasone, 40 mg/d orally on Days 1 through 4, 9 through 12, and 17 through 20. Thalidomide is also an effective drug in patients with myeloma that is refractory to conventional therapy. Other forms of supportive care for patients with myeloma include local radiotherapy to painful bony sites, recombinant erythropoietin, and appropriate antibiotics when the need arises.

Amyloidosis

Approximately 10% of all patients with multiple myeloma develop amyloidosis (primary amyloidosis). Conversely, in 60% of all patients with amyloidosis, the amyloid protein is light-chained derived and there is a coexistent proliferation of plasma cells in the bone marrow cavity that may overlap the features of myeloma. Primary amyloidosis (AL) is treated in the same manner as stage I myeloma. Likewise, amyloidosis-complicating myeloma is treated based on the stage of the myeloma.

Solitary Plasmacytoma of Bone

Patients with a solitary plasmacytoma of bone actually have stage I myeloma, and given enough time, the myeloma will become clinically overt in most patients. Local radiotherapy is the appropriate treatment for patients with solitary plasmacytoma of bone. Melphalan and prednisone can be withheld until symptoms develop (usually about 24 months). Patients with extramedullay plasmacytoma (the usual site is typically the nasal cavity) do not have myeloma. Rather, such patients have a potentially curable malignancy, and the treatment is local radiotherapy to the involved area.

Other Lymphoproliferative Disorders

Hairy cell leukemia (HCL) is a rare malignancy of unknown cause that clinically can be confused with malignant lymphomas such as splenic lymphoma with villous lymphocytes, CLL, and other low-grade NHL. The symptoms of HCL include malaise, fatigue, and recurrent bacterial infections including tuberculosis. The clinical findings are splenomegally and pancytopenia. The diagnosis relies on a bone marrow aspirate and biopsy with the demonstration of tartrate resistant acid phosphatase within the hairy cells. Treatment of HCL consists of either cladribine or pentostatin.

Waldenström macroglobulinemia represents a forme fruste of malignant lymphoma, diffuse small lymphocytic that oversynthesizes a monoclonal IgM paraprotein. The circulating IgM can lead to hyperviscosity, cryoglobulinemia, cold agglutinin hemolytic anemia, peripheral neuropathy, glomerular disease, and amyloidosis (when the IgM is deposited in tissues). The symptoms of hyperviscosity include visual disturbances, dizziness, lethargy, bleeding disorders, or neuropathy. The diagnosis is made based on the presence of a monoclonal IgM and the results of a bone marrow aspirate and biopsy or lymph node biopsy showing the presence of plasmacytoid lymphocytes, which are indistinguishable from the small lymphocytes characteristic of CLL or NHL, diffuse small lymphocytic. The treatment of Waldenström macroblobulinemia consists of plasmapheresis followed by either fludarabine or cladribine. The median survival of patients with Waldenström macroglobulinemia is 5 to 7 years.

Heavy-chain diseases are all lymphoproliferative disorders characterized by the overproduction of an incomplete immunoglobulin molecule that lacks light chains. Alpha (incomplete IgA) or gamma (incomplete IgG) heavy-chain disease presents and behaves like an NHL, and both are treated as such. Alpha heavy-chain disease (Mediterranean lymphoma) represents an NHL with a predilection for abdominal and small bowel involvement. Gamma heavy-chain disease represents an NHL with a predilection for hepatic and splenic involvement, involvement of Waldeyer ring, eosinophilia, leukopenia, and thrombocytopenia. Mu heavy-chain disease (incomplete IgM) is associated exclusively with CLL.

Post-transplantation lymphoproliferative disease is a polyclonal disorder that arises in patients who have undergone a solid organ transplant while receiving immunosuppressive therapy. This lymphoproliferative disorder is associated with Epstein-Barr viral infection. The clinical manifestations are progressive lymphadenopathy. In most instances, if immunosuppressive drugs are reduced or temporarily withdrawn, the lymphadenopathy regresses.

Large granular lymphocytic leukemia (LGLL), also known as T-cell lymphocytosis with cytopenia, is a rare disease characterized by a proliferation of large granular lymphocytes. The neutropenia associated with LGLL may be cyclic, and the anemia is most consistent with pure red cell aplasia. Large granular lymphocytic leukemia is associated with rheumatoid arthritis, and many patients have been diagnosed with Felty syndrome. The course of LGLL is usually benign and rarely requires cytotoxic therapy.

Chapter 8

Myeloid Neoplasia

.

Acute Myeloid Leukemia

Acute myeloid leukemia (AML) is a malignant neoplasm of a committed myeloid progenitor cell. In 2000, an estimated 18,000 adults will develop AML. The etiology of AML is unknown; however, both an increased incidence of myelodysplasia and AML have been reported to occur in persons who have had prolonged exposure to benzene and/or petroleum products. Other etiologic agents include alkylating agents (melphalan, cyclophosphamide, mechlorethamine), topoisomerase II inhibitors (etoposide), anthracyclines (doxorubicin), anthracenediones (mitoxantrone), azathioprine, and chlorambucil. Immunologic disorders such as ataxia-telangiectasia, Wiskott-Aldrich syndrome, and X-linked agammaglobulinemia are also associated with an increased incidence of AML.

Symptoms and Signs

Patients with AML exhibit signs and symptoms of fatigue, easy bruisability or bleeding, fever, and infection. The physical findings may be minimal or may include pallor, ecchymosis, or petechiae. The laboratory findings usually demonstrate a low or elevated leukocyte count, with anemia and thrombocytopenia. Hyperuricemia may be present. In patients with acute promyelocytic leukemia (APL) disseminated intravascular coagulation is commonplace.

Treatment and Prognosis

The French-American-British (FAB) subtypes of AML and the cytogenetic abnormalities observed are listed in Tables 8-1 and 8-2. The cytogenetic abnormalities confer prognostic information. For example, M2 with t(8;21), M3, and M4 with an inversion 16 all carry very favorable prognoses with high complete remission (CR) rates and a good probability of a curative outcome. Such patients are not candidates for allogeneic bone marrow transplantation in first CR.

The treatment of AML consists of induction therapy designed to reduce the leukemic burden rapidly so that it is undetected by light microscopy followed by consolidative therapy that further serves to decrease the leukemic burden theoretically to zero. A popular treatment regimen is shown in Figure 8-1. Typically, on the fourteenth day after induction therapy, a bone marrow aspirate is performed to determine the presence of any residual leukemic cells. If blasts are present, additional chemotherapy with high-dose cytosine arabinoside (HI-DAC) 3000 mg/m^2 given intravenously over 2 hours every 12 hours for six doses is administered. If the bone marrow is "empty," the patient is supported with antibiotics and blood products (see Chapter 5, p 95) until hematologic recovery takes place and then consolidation therapy is administered.

The exception to this generalization is patients with APL [APL, FAB M3, t(15;17)]. These patients have an altered retinoic acid receptor (rar) α gene

Table 8-1 Chromosomal Abnormalities Associated with Acute Myeloid Leukemia

Neoplasm	Genes	Chromosomal Abnormalities
Acute myeloid leukemia		
with maturation		t(8;21)
with basophilia	PEK/CAN	t(6;9)

Table 8-2 French-American-British (FAB) Subtypes of Acute Myeloid Leukemia

FAB Classification	Chromosomal Abnormalities
M0: Undifferentiated	11q13
M1: Myeloid	−5, −7, −17, del 3p, +21, +8
M2: Myeloid with differentiation	t(8;21), inv3, −5, −7, t(6;9), +8
M3: Promyelocytic	t:15;17
M4: Myelomonocytic	inv16, −16q, t(8;21), −5,−7, t(6;9)
M5: Monocytic	t(9;11), +8
M6: Erythroid	−5q, −5, −7, −3, +8
M7: Megakaryocytic	+8, +21, inv or del 13

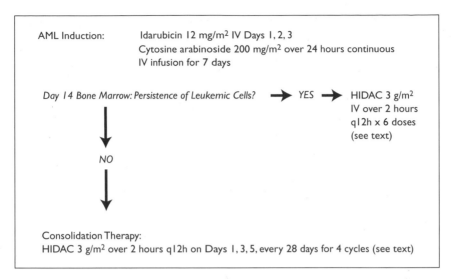

AML Induction: Idarubicin 12 mg/m² IV Days 1, 2, 3
                      Cytosine arabinoside 200 mg/m² over 24 hours continuous
                      IV infusion for 7 days

Day 14 Bone Marrow: Persistence of Leukemic Cells? ➡ YES ➡ HIDAC 3 g/m²
                                                               IV over 2 hours
                                                               q12h x 6 doses
                                                               (see text)

                      NO

Consolidation Therapy:
HIDAC 3 g/m² over 2 hours q12h on Days 1, 3, 5, every 28 days for 4 cycles (see text)

Figure 8-1 Treatment regimen for acute myeloid leukemia. HIDAC = high-dose cytosine arabinoside.

that synthesizes an altered rar-α. Patients with APL should first be given a course of all-*trans*-retinoic acid (ATRA) 45 mg/m² orally daily in two divided doses for a minimum of 45 days to a maximum of 90 days. The ATRA induces differentiation of the APL cells; however, remissions with ATRA alone are of short duration (median, 3.5 months). In 25% of patients with APL treated with ATRA a "retinoic acid syndrome" develops, consisting of fever, respiratory distress with pulmonary infiltrates, pseudotumor cerebri, pleural effusions, or cardiovascular collapse. Treatment of the retinoic acid syndrome consists of discontinuing ATRA and using high-dose steroids and either hydroxyurea or conventional therapy to control the leukocytosis. Although the induction chemotherapy for patients with APL is identical to that shown in Figure 8-1, the consolidation therapy is limited to only two cycles. Consolidation 1 consists of another round of induction therapy; Consolidation 2 is HIDAC at 1000 mg/m² over 2 hours every 12 hours for eight doses and daunorubicin at 45 mg/m² IVP on Days 1 through 4. Most recently, arsenic trioxide has been shown to be highly active in patients with APL.

After hematologic recovery manifests itself, a repeat bone marrow is done to document a CR. It is obvious that a CR is the first step in a curative outcome. The roles of autologous (ABMT) and allogeneic (alloBMT) bone marrow transplantation have recently been tested in a randomized clinical trial in patients with AML in first CR (1). This trial showed no survival benefit overall for ABMT or alloBMT. However, alloBMT may still have a role in certain subsets of patients with AML. Thus, the need for additional therapy such as

Table 8-3 Median Survial and Probability of Disease-Free Survival at 5 Years as a Function of the French-American-British (FAB) Classification and Cytogenetic Abnormalities

FAB	Median Survival (mo)	5-year Disease-Free Survival (%)
M0 with 11q23	<6	0
M1 with −5, −7	8	20
M1 with +8	15	30
M2 with t(8;21)	24	40
M2 with −5, −7	8	20
M3 with t(15,17)	>60	60–79
M4 with inv 16	>60	65
M4 with t(8;21)	24	40
M4 with −5, −7	8	20
M5 with t(9;11) or +8	15	30
M6 with −5, −7	8	20
M6 with +8	15	30
M7 with +8, +21	15–18	30–40

alloBMT is determined by the type of leukemia, FAB classification (see Table 8-2), and the cytogenetic abnormality that is present. As shown in Table 8-3, some patients with AML have favorable or intermediate prognosis, and accordingly alloBMT is unnecessary. These patients are those with APL, AML-FAB M4 with inversion 16, and M1, M2, M5 +8, or M4 with t(8;21). Other patients clearly have exceedingly poor prognoses. Patients with FAB M0 or patients with abnormalities of chromosomes 5 and 7 are candidates for alloBMT in first CR. Patients with favorable or intermediate prognosis AML who experience relapse are candidates for alloBMT.

Elderly patients (55 to 70 years old) with AML should receive GM-CSF (sargramostim [Leukine]) 5 µg/kg/d after induction therapy/chemotherapy to shorten the duration of neutropenia, thereby decreasing treatment-related mortality.

Treatment of Refractory or Relapsed Acute Myeloid Leukemia

Patients who fail to achieve a CR after two courses of induction have a grim prognosis. Such patients are candidates for clinical trials using experimental therapies, because conventional chemotherapy using either single agents or combinations tends to produce limited results. The current generation of clinical trials is examining monoclonal antibodies directed against myeloid leukemia cells. Patients younger than 55 years old who achieve CR but then experience relapse should receive chemotherapy with an attempt to have them attain a second CR; if an allogeneic bone marrow donor is available for these patients, an alloBMT should also be performed. Useful chemotherapy regimens for relapsed AML include high-dose cytosine arabinoside in combination with mitoxantrone, etoposide, idarubicin, or fludarabine. These two combinations produce short-lived CRs (duration 4 to 6 months) in 40% to 60% of patients.

In patients who are in first relapse or in second CR, alloBMT results in a 30% to 40% disease-free survival rate in 5 years. Autologous bone marrow transplants are an option in patients younger than 65 years of age for whom an allogeneic bone marrow donor is not available; however, the results are inferior to those of alloBMTs, with 20% to 30% of patients alive and disease-free at 5 years. The explanation for these inferior results is that with autologous bone marrow transplants there is no graft versus leukemia effect.

Currently there are ongoing studies in AML to examine better and more effective modes of therapy; this underscores the need to encourage patients with AML to enroll in clinical trials.

Chronic Myelogenous Leukemia

Chronic myelogenous leukemia (CML) is a clonal disorder that results from neoplastic transformation of a primitive uncommitted bone marrow stem cell. This uncommitted bone marrow cell has the capacity to commit to myeloid, erythroid, lymphoid, monocytic, and megakaryocytic cell lineage; however, bone marrow stromal cells are uninvolved. Although the cause of CML remains unknown; the molecular basis of CML is a result of a balanced translocation between the long arms of chromosomes 9 and 22, t(9;22) (q43, q11), the Philadelphia chromosome (see Chapter 1, p 15). This balanced translocation results in a fusion gene that encodes for a mutant protein with a molecular weight of 210 kD that begins with the amino acid sequence of the c-*abl* oncogene and terminates with the amino acid sequence of *bcr*. This mutant protein has a markedly increased autophosphorylating activity and can transform transfected cells and can induce leukemia in transgeneic mice.

Symptoms and Signs

Chronic myelogenous leukemia is a disease process that is seen in all age groups; however, the median age of presentation is 50 years. There is a slight male predominance. The presenting signs are fatigue, weight loss, and left upper quadrant pain. In patients with leukocyte counts of more than 100,000/mm^3, the symptoms may include those of hyperviscosity, which include priapism, tinnitus, stupor, or cerebrovascular accidents. The laboratory data show an elevated leukocyte count, usually greater than 25,000 cell/μL. The differential usually shows granulocytes in all stages of maturation from mature polymorphonuclear leukocytes to blasts. Basophils are elevated greater than 4% by usually less than 7% of the total white blood cell count. The platelet count is elevated in 30% to 50% of patients with CML.

The bone marrow in patients with CML is hypercellular with a myeloid/erythoid ratio of 10–30/1. Myelocytes are the dominant cells, with blasts and promyelocytes accounting for fewer than 10% of the cells. The megakaryocytes may show some evidence of dysplasia, and an increase in stromal reticulin may be present.

Other laboratory findings include a reduced leukocyte alkaline phosphatase score, an elevated transcobalamin (vitamin B_{12}) level, and increased lactate dehydrogenase and uric acid levels. The diagnosis of CML is based on the peripheral smear and bone marrow examination. The differential diagnosis is a leukemoid reaction. Usually the distinction between CML and a leukemoid reaction is relatively clear, as shown in Table 8-4. Bone marrow cytogenetics should be performed. The presence of the balanced translocation between chromosomes 9 and 22 confirms the diagnosis of CML; however, the Philadelphia chromosome is present in only 90% to 95% of patients with CML. The absence of a Philadelphia chromosome does not in any way negate a diagnosis of CML if the other features of the disease are present.

Treatment and Prognosis

Patients with CML have a clinical course that is defined by phases of the disease process. Most patients are diagnosed with CML in chronic phase. Patients in chronic phase are either asymptomatic or experience fatigue or malaise. The peripheral smear shows a small percentage of blasts and promyelocytes (<10%). In accelerated phase, patients usually are more symptomatic and are likely to experience fever, night sweats, or weight loss. The peripheral smear usually shows 15% to 30% blasts or more than 30% blasts and promyelocytes.

The blastic phase of CML resembles an acute leukemia. Patients in blast phase are symptomatic with weight loss, fever, night sweats, and bone pain. The physical findings may show pallor, lymphadenopathy, and, sometimes, subcutaneous nodules. The diagnosis of blast-phase CML is made when bone marrow examination reveals more than 30% blasts.

The treatment of CML depends on the age of the patient and the availability of a human leukocyte antigen (HLA)–matched bone marrow donor, because the only *curative* therapy is alloBMT. The results of alloBMT are best when patients undergo transplantation during chronic phase. The results of transplantation in accelerated or blast phase are inferior (Table 8-5). Patients who experience relapse with CML after alloBMT can be treated with donor lymphocyte infusions (DLI), which in 70% to 80% of patients who have had relapse with CML can result in a histologic and cytogenetic remission. The rationale for DLI is that these donor lymphocytes can re-establish a graft-versus-leukemia effect. Obviously, the danger of DLI is graft-versus-host disease.

Most patients with CML do not have an HLA-matched bone marrow donor or are older than age 55 years. In such patients, the best treatment is a combina-

Table 8-4 Distinction Between Chronic Myelogenous Leukemia (CML) and Leukemoid Reaction

Findings	CML	Leukemoid Reaction
Physical Findings		
Splenic enlargement	+	—
Laboratory Findings		
Increased WBC	+	+
Blasts and promyelocytes	+	—
LAP	Decreased	Normal
Transcobalamin	Increased	Normal
LDH	Increased	Normal

LAP = leukocyte alkaline phosphatase; LDH = lactate dehydrogenase.

Table 8-5 Results of Allogenic Bone Marrow Transplantation in Chronic Myelogenous Leukemia

Phase	Disease-Free Survival (%)	Survival (15- and 20-year) (%)
Chronic	50–70	50–80
Accelerated	30–40	30–40
Blastic	10–20	10–20

tion of interferon 5×10^6 U/m^2/d and hydroxyurea. Hematologic remission (defined as a normalization of the complete blood count) with this combination usually occurs within the first 2 months of therapy. Cytogenetic remission, which is defined as a disappearance or decrease in the number of Philadelphia chromosome–bearing cells, takes longer to achieve. The response to interferon and hydroxyurea is dependent on the phase during which treatment is started. The combination is most effective in patients in chronic phase. Patients in blastic phase respond poorly to therapy and have a limited survival.

Myeloproliferative Disorders

Polycythemia rubra vera (PRV) is a clonal proliferation of a primitive hematopoietic stem cell that results in an uncontrolled growth of erythroid progenitors and mature erythrocytes. Polycythemia rubra vera is similar to CML in the sense that it too is a clonal process of an uncommitted bone marrow stem cell; however, in PRV, unlike CML, a unique cytogenetic abnormality has not been found.

Polycythemia rubra vera is a rare disease (2500 to 2700 cases annually) with a male predominance and usually occurs in the fifth to sixth decades of life; it is uncommon in patients younger than 40 years old.

Symptoms and Signs

The symptoms of this disease are a result of an increased hematocrit that leads to turbulent blood flow, which in turn leads to vascular occlusive episodes. The presenting symptoms are nonspecific and include headaches, weakness, pruritus, dizziness, sweats, paresthesias, visual disturbances, epigastric distress, and weight loss. The physical findings include a ruddy complexion, conjunctival plethora, splenomegaly, hepatomegaly, and hypertension. Patients with PRV are at risk for thromboses and hemorrhage. Thromboses may occur in the venous system of the lower extremities, pulmonary embolism, and arterial occlusions in the coronary and peripheral vascular system. Patients with PRV are at risk for Budd-Chiari syndrome (hepatic vein or inferior vena cava thrombosis [hepatosplenomegaly, ascites, lower extremity edema, jaundice, abdominal pain]) and portal vein thrombosis (ascites, splenomegaly).

The laboratory findings show an increased hematocrit level, leukocytosis, and thrombocytosis. The work-up includes obtaining a red cell mass, serum erythropoietin level, and oxygen saturation. The diagnostic criteria for PRV are shown in Table 8-6. These laboratory tests discriminate PRV from secondary erythrocytosis and spurious erythrocytosis (hemoconcentration secondary to dehydration, hypersplenism, pre-eclampsia, pheochromocytoma, carbon monoxide intoxication) (Table 8-7). A bone marrow examination is necessary in PRV to confirm the diagnosis and to conduct cytogenetic analysis. The most common cytogenetic abnormalities are trisomy of chromosomes 8 and 9 and the deletion of the long arm of chromosome 20 (20q).

Table 8-6 Clinical and Laboratory Criteria for Polycythemia Rubra Vera

Increased red cell mass (>36 mL/kg for men; >32 mL/kg women)
Normal oxygen saturation (>92%)
Splenomegaly
Thrombocytosis (>400,000 platelets/μL) and leukocytosis (>12,000 cells/μL)
Bone marrow hypercellularity with megakaryocytic hyperplasia; absent iron stores
Low serum erythropoietin levels

Table 8-7 Differential Diagnosis of Polycythemia Rubra Vera (PRV)

Findings	PRV	Secondary Erythrocytosis	Spurious Erythrocytosis
Red cell mass	Increased	Increased	Normal
O_2 saturation	Normal	Decreased	Normal
Serum erythropoietin levels	Low	Increased	Normal

Treatment and Prognosis

The preferred treatment of PRV is phlebotomy, unless there is coexistent thrombocytosis (platelets >400,000/μL). Allopurinol, 300 mg, should be used to control the hyperuricemia.

In the absence of thrombocytosis, the goal of phlebotomy is to decrease the hematocrit to 45%, thereby significantly decreasing the incidence of thrombotic/hemorrhagic complications. A 1- to 2-U phlebotomy, no more frequently than every other day or twice weekly in patients with cardiovascular disease, should decrease the hematocrit to 45%. Periodic monthly phlebotomy may be required to maintain the hematocrit at this level. If thrombocytosis is present, a chemotherapeutic agent is initially used to decrease the platelet count before phlebotomy. Hydroxyurea is an excellent drug to use in this setting. The initial dose is 2000 mg/d for 1 week followed by 1000 to 1500 mg/d until the platelet count is less than 300,000/μL. Hydroxyurea is sufficiently myelosuppressive that phlebotomy may not be required. Another alternative is anagrelide, which is initially dosed at 0.5 mg orally four times daily with increments of 0.5 mg/d until the platelet count is less than 300,000/μL. Anagrelide should be used with caution in patients with cardiovascular disease because of its toxicities, which include vasodilatation, fluid retention, congestive heart failure, palpitations, and tachycardia. Other toxicities include nausea, headaches, and dizziness. Phlebotomy is usually done after administration of anagrelide, with the goal of decreasing the hematocrit to 45%. If such measures fail, other agents such as interferon, busulfan, or P32 can be used.

Polycythemia rubra vera usually carries a favorable prognosis. If patients receive optimal treatment, the median survival is 10 to 15 years. Some patients with PRV have an aggressive course. Approximately 10% to 15% of patients with PRV develop postpolycythemic myeloid metaplasia (PPMM), which represents the spent or fibrotic phase of PRV. In these patients, a clinical picture of cytopenias, myelofibrosis, and extramedullary hematopoiesis develops. Platelet-derived growth factor may be responsible for this transformation. Patients with PPMM are at high risk for acute leukemia, and the median survival is 6.5 years.

Primary Thrombocythemia

Primary thrombocythemia (PT) is a myeloproliferative disorder that leads to the sustained and unregulated proliferation of megakaryocytes, which in turn results in chronic thrombocytosis (platelets >600,000/μL). Like PRV, PT is a rare disease, accounting for no more than 1500 to 2000 cases annually. It is a disease of middle age, most often occurring between 50 and 60 years of age, and the number of men and women affected is equal. The cause of PT is un-

Table 8-8 Diagnostic Criteria for Primary Thrombocythemia

Platelet count >600,000/μL on two different occasions 1 month apart
Absence of infection, inflammation, or nonhematologic malignancy
Splenomegaly
Absence of marrow fibrosis
Absence of Philadelphia chromosome
Absence of iron deficiency
Normal red cell mass

known; however, like all myeloproliferative disorders, the disease is derived from a clonal stem cell process. Thrombopoietin levels are usually low in PT.

Symptoms and Signs

The clinical manifestations are thromboembolic complications either in the microcirculation of the extremities and in the central nervous system or in the large arteries of the lower extremities. The physical findings may include gangrenous changes in the fingertips and toes, acrocyanosis, splenomegaly (50% of patients), and hepatomegaly (20% of patients). In most patients, the laboratory findings demonstrate thrombocytosis (>600,000 cells/μL; sometimes >1,000,000/μL) and a normal hemoglobin level. Approximately one fourth of patients may be mildly anemic.

The diagnostic criteria for PT are listed in Table 8-8, and the differential diagnosis includes secondary thrombocytosis and iron deficiency. The bone marrow examination demonstrates hypercellularity, an increase in megakaryocytes with aggregates of megakaryocytes and atypical forms, micromegakaryocytes, and dysplastic changes in the megakaryocytic nuclei.

Treatment and Prognosis

The treatment of PT consists of anagrelide 0.5 mg orally four times daily for 1 week with the dose adjusted by 0.5 mg/d every 7 days until the platelet count is less than 450,000/μL. An alternative treatment is hydroxyurea, starting at 1000 mg/d and adjusting the dose until the platelet count is less than 450,000/μL. In patients refractory to or intolerant of anagrelide or hydroxyurea, interferon-α is used. Patients with PT have a favorable overall prognosis; the 10-year survival exceeds 75%.

Agnogenic Myeloid Metaplasia

Agnogenic myeloid metaplasia (AMM) is a malignant disorder characterized by bone marrow fibrosis, extramedullary hematopoiesis, splenomegaly, and a

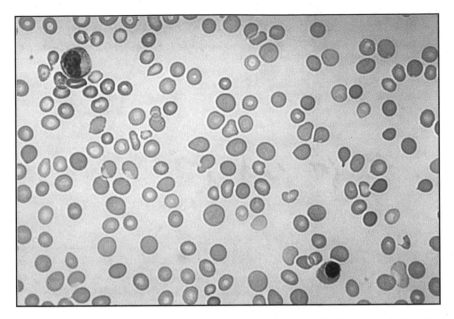

Figure 8-2 Peripheral smear of a patient with agnogenic myeloid metaplasia. A nucleated red blood cell is seen in the lower right-hand corner; teardrop forms are scattered throughout the smear (×400).

peripheral blood smear that shows a leukoerythroblastic picture with tear drop forms of erythrocytes (Fig. 8-2). In AMM, the bone marrow fibrosis is believed to occur in response to a clonal proliferation of hematopoietic stem cells that ultimately leads to bone marrow failure; however, what clonal proliferative process should provoke marrow fibrosis and why is as yet poorly understood. Agnogenic myeloid metaplasia is an exceedingly rare disease, with major referral centers seeing on average only 5 to 10 patients per year.

Symptoms and Signs

The average age of patients with AMM is 60 years, and the presenting symptoms are fatigue, weight loss, night sweats, early satiety (splenomegaly). The physical findings in patients with AMM include pallor, splenomegaly, hepatomegaly, and, rarely, portal hypertension. The laboratory findings show anemia (ineffective erythropoiesis and splenic sequestration). The anemia is normochromic/normocytic but can be hypochromic/microcytic owing to occult blood loss. In addition to the anemia, leukocytosis or leukopenia, thrombocytopenia, or, rarely, thrombocytosis may be present. The smear shows a classic leukoerythroblastic picture (see Fig. 8-2). The diagnosis relies on a bone marrow aspirate that typically results in a "dry tap" and prompts a bone marrow biopsy. The differential diagnosis of AMM is shown in Table 8-9.

Table 8-9 Differential Diagnosis of Agnogenic Myeloid Metaplasia

Disseminated tuberculosis or histoplasmosis
Hairy cell leukemia
Postpolycythemic myeloid metaplasia/chronic myelogenous leukemia
Acute myelofibrosis

The bone marrow biopsy differentiates tuberculosis or histoplasmosis from AMM by the presence of granulomas; hairy cell leukemia has a distinctive biopsy appearance and is readily diagnosed. The marrow in acute myelofibrosis—a misnomer because it is actually a form of acute megakaryocytic leukemia (FAB M7)—shows the presence of blasts that express megakaryocytic markers. Finally, the distinction between postpolycythemic myeloid metaplasia and CML is impossible to make unless there is a previous history.

Treatment and Prognosis

Agnogenic myeloid metaplasia is an incurable disease, and the treatment approach is palliative. No "standard therapy" exists for this disease. Younger patients (<55 years old) who have an HLA-matched related donor should be offered alloBMT. In patients who are older or for whom a marrow donor is not available, treatment should be focused on relief of symptoms. For example, hydroxyurea can palliate the pressure-like symptoms of splenomegaly. Patients with AMM and a hypermetabolic syndrome (weight loss, diarrhea, and cachexia) can be palliated with steroids. Patients with enlarged and painful spleens or those with thrombocytopenia or hemolytic anemia as a result of splenic sequestration may receive radiation therapy to the spleen. In my judgment, splenectomy should rarely if ever be performed in patients with AMM because it accelerates the transformation to M7 leukemia (see section on acute myeloid leukemia earlier in this chapter). The median survival of patients with AMM is 3 to 4 years.

Myelodysplasia

Myelodysplasia (MDS) defines a grouping of clonal hematologic disorders that are characterized clinically and morphologically by ineffective hematopoiesis. The infective hematopoiesis reflects itself by the presence of refractory cytopenias (usually anemia with or without thrombocytopenia) and morphologic dysplastic changes in the bone marrow involving at least one of the three hematopoietic lineages. Like the other myeloproliferative disorders described in this chapter, myelodysplasia is a clonal disorder involving a com-

Table 8-10 Classification of Myelodysplasia

Myelodysplasia	Bone Marrow Blasts	Sideroblasts
Refractory anemia	<5%	Absent
Refractory anemia with ringed sideroblasts	<5%	Present
Refractory anemia with excess blasts	5–20	Absent/present
Chronic myelomonocytic leukemia	≤20	Absent/present
Refractory anemia with excess blasts in transformation	21–30	Absent/present

mitted myeloid stem cell. Some patients with MDS may have an indolent course; for most patients with MDS, the disease eventually evolves into acute myeloid leukemia.

The classification of MDS is shown in Table 8-10. Myelodysplasia is a grouping of five distinct clinical entities that are characterized by ineffective hematopoiesis as a result of an uncoupling of the normally orderly process of proliferation and differentiation. In other words, what seems to characterize the hematopoietic progenitors of patients with MDS, at least in vitro, is their ability to respond to proliferative growth factors but their inability to stop proliferating when exposed to inhibitory hematopoietic factors or bone marrow factors that promote the differentiation process. At present, it is unclear whether this defect occurs as a result of a defective cell membrane receptor or abnormal signal transduction.

The introduction of the FAB classification of MDS has provided a benchmark for uniform nomenclature and diagnostic criteria; however, critics correctly point out that the term "refractory anemia" is imprecise and cannot be identified morphologically. Similarly, chronic myelomonocytic leukemia (CMMoL) is more closely related to the myeloproliferative syndromes than MDS. Finally, the FAB classification correlates roughly with prognosis.

The International Myelodysplastic Syndrome Risk Analysis Workshop has proposed the International Prognostic Scoring System for MDS, which seems to correlate well with survival (Table 8-11).

Clonal cytogenetic abnormalities are characteristic of MDS. These abnormalities include 5q–, monosomy 7, trisomy 8, monosomy 5, 20q–, loss of an X or Y, and t(5;7) (treatment-related MDS). Some chromosomal abnormalities occur more frequently in certain subtypes of MDS. For example, patients with refractory anemia typically have a 5q–. Patients with the 5q– syndrome tend to have an indolent clinical course, and because the principal treatment is erythrocyte transfusions, these patients are at high risk for iron overload. Patients with CMMoL most often have 20q– abnormalities.

Table 8-11 International Prognostic Scoring System for Myelodysplasia

Blasts (%)	Cytogenetics	Cytopenia*	Score
<5	Normal, Y–, 5q–, 20q–	None or one	0
5–10	All others	Two or three	0.5
11–20	Abnormal 7, or 3 or more		1.0
21–30			1.5

Overall Score	Median survival (years)
Low: 0	5.7
Intermediate	
0.5–1.0	3.5
1.5–2.0	1.2
High: ≥2.5	0.4

*Cytopenia = Hgb <10 g/dL, ANC <1500, platelets <100,000/μL.
Republished with permission from Heaney ML, Golde DW. Myelodysplasia. N Engl J Med. 1999;340:1649-60.

Patients with therapy-related MDS may have t(5;7) or balanced translocations involving chromosomes 3q26, 11q23, or 21q22. These patients have a grim prognosis.

Symptoms and Signs

Myelodysplasia is a disease of the elderly (median age >60 years) unless it is treatment related. The incidence of MDS in the population older than 70 years old is 22 to 45 cases per 100,000 persons. The symptoms of MDS are fatigue, recurrent infections, or bleeding. The physical findings in MDS are not dramatic and include pallor petechiae. The laboratory findings are usually anemia, thrombocytopenia, monocytosis, neutropenia, or some combination of these. The presence of such unexplained laboratory findings is what should raise the suspicion of MDS.

Ultimately, the diagnosis of MDS relies on the bone marrow and cytogenetic findings. The bone marrow aspirate is hypercellular with dysmyelopoietic (dysplastic) changes in the erythroid, myeloid, and megakaryocytic lineages (Fig. 8-3). The morphologic changes in MDS are asynchronous nuclear/cytoplasmic maturation in the myeloid and erythroid series, abnormal megakaryocytes that may be small in size (micromegakaryocytes) or that may have only one nucleus. A small number of patients with MDS may have a hypocellular marrow or show fibrotic marrow changes. The bone marrow of patients with refractory anemia with ringed sideroblasts (RARS) shows dysmyelopoietic changes in the erythroid series and ringed sideroblasts, which

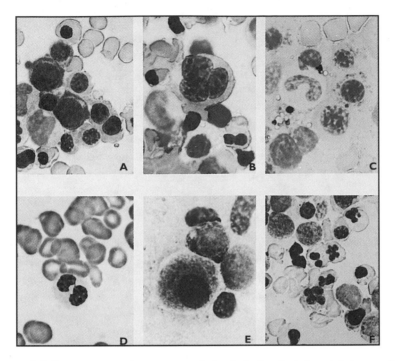

Figure 8-3 Bone marrow changes in myelodysplasia. Panels A, B, and F show various dysmyelopoietic changes (megaloblastoid) in the erythroid lineage. Panel C is an iron stain of a marrow with refractory sideroblastic anemia and shows the typical perinuclear deposition of iron. Panel D is of a granulocyte with a Pelger-Huët abnormality. Panel E shows a micromegakaryocyte (×200). (Republished with permission from Heaney ML, Golde DW. Myelodysplasia. N Engl J Med. 1999;340:1649-60.)

are iron granules that ring at least one third of the nuclear circumference. The bone marrow of patients with CMMoL has an increase in monocytes in addition to the dysmyelopoietic changes. It is based on the marrow findings that the subtype of MDS is defined.

Treatment and Prognosis

In most patients, the treatment of MDS is supportive. Younger patients with MDS are candidates for alloBMT, provided that an HLA-compatible related donor is available.

Most patients with MDS are supported with erythrocyte transfusions, platelet transfusions, and for patients with neutropenia or recurrent infections, filgrastim or sargramostim. Recombinant human erythropoietin has a limited role in MDS; only 25% of patients respond to it. Combinations of erythropoietin and filgrastim stimulate erythropoiesis in 38% to 48% of patients with MDS. Low-dose cytosine arabinoside may be an option in some patients.

The course of MDS is highly variable. Some patients with MDS (those with refractory anemia or RARS with normal cytogenetic findings) may remain stable for many years before the disease transforms into acute leukemia (see Table 8-11). Patients with CMMoL can survive for years before leukemic transformation (myelomonocytic) occurs. In patients with refractory anemia with excess blasts or refractory anemia with excess blasts in transformation and cytogenetic abnormalities, transformation into acute leukemia usually occurs within 18 months.

REFERENCE

1. **Cassileth PA, Harrington DP, Appelbaum FR, et al.** Chemotherapy compared with autologous or allogeneic bone marrow transplantation in the management of acute myeloid leukemia in first remission. N Engl J Med. 1998;339:1649-56.

Chapter 9

Head and Neck and
Thoracic Malignancies

Head and Neck Cancers

Head and neck cancers are a diverse group of relatively uncommon tumors. Head and neck cancers account for 2% to 3% of all cancers in the United States. Patients who are diagnosed with these cancers are at risk to develop thoracic malignancies, such as lung or esophageal cancer. Head and neck cancers are more common among men than women and typically occur between 50 and 70 years of age. The risk factors include tobacco smoking as well as the use of smokeless tobacco, alcohol, occupational exposure (wood dust [nasopharyngeal], nickel, radiation exposure, and the Epstein-Barr virus [nasopharyngeal]).

Symptoms and Signs

The symptoms of head and neck cancer vary with their location but generally include alterations in swallowing, phonation, hearing, and respiration. Cancers of the mouth cause pain, dysphagia, odynophagia, and alterations in speech. Laryngeal cancers produce hoarseness and hemoptysis. Nasopharyngeal cancers cause hemoptysis, stuffiness of the ear, and trismus. Only occasionally the primary site provokes a few symptoms and the presenting complaint is a "lump in the neck" that reflects the nodal metastasis.

The physical findings vary with the primary site. Cancers of the oral cavity usually cause an indurated and/or ulcerated mass in the tongue, floor of the mouth, buccal mucosa, or lip. Cancer of the base of the tongue is notoriously infiltrative into muscle and is only discovered by palpation. Cancer of the tonsillar pillar causes pain, and on examination a tonsillar mass is found. Cancers of the hypopharynx, larynx, and nasopharynx require indirect or direct endoscopy (referral to an ENT specialist) ultimately to establish a diagnosis in that location.

After a diagnosis of a head and neck cancer has been established, the patient is staged and, on the basis of staging, treatment decisions are made (Table 9-1).

Treatment and Prognosis

The treatment of head and neck cancer varies with the anatomic site and stage. Stage I and II cancers of the anterior two thirds of the tongue can be adequately treated with radiotherapy alone (60–70 Gy/6–7 weeks), with a resultant disease-free survival at 5 years of 80% to 85% for stage I and 60% to 75% for stage II. Patients with stage III or IV disease are treated with either a glossectomy or

Table 9-1 Staging of Head and Neck Cancer

Tumor

T0	Carcinoma in situ
T1	Tumor <2 cm or confined to a regional anatomic site
T2	Tumor >2 cm <4 cm or tumor extending to adjacent anatomic region
T3	Tumor >4 cm and extending into adjacent region; if larynx, fixed vocal cord involvement
T4	Tumor with deep invasion (i.e, bone skin or cartilage)

Nodes

N0	No clinical regional nodal involvement
N1	Ipsilateral node <3 cm
N2	
N2A	Single ipsilateral node >3 cm <6 cm
N2B	Multiple ipsilateral nodes <6 cm
N2C	Bilateral nodes
N3	Lymph nodes >6 cm

Metastases

M0	No distant metastases
M1	Distant metastases present

Stage Groupings

Stage 0	T0, N0, M0
Stage I	T1, N0, M0
Stage II	T2, N0, M0
Stage III	T3, N0, M0; or T1-3, N1, M0
Stage IV	T4, N0, M0; or any T, N2 or N3, M0; or any T, any N, M1

composite resection and postoperative radiotherapy to the neck for stage III/IV patients with no regional nodal involvement (N0). Radical neck dissection is reserved for patients with nodal involvement (N1–3). The 5-year survival for patients with stage III and stage IV cancer is 66% and 30% to 35%, respectively.

The treatment of nasopharyngeal cancer is radiation therapy (65–70 Gy) to the primary tumor and the draining lymph nodes and concurrent chemotherapy such as 5-fluorouracil (5-FU) and cisplatin or cisplatin and paclitaxel (Taxol). Surgical resection is never attempted. Because most patients present with stage III or IV disease, the overall 5-year survival is 50%.

Oropharyngeal cancers, cancers of the base of the tongue, tonsil, and tonsillar pillar, are treated in a manner similar to that of cancers of the oral cavity: radiation therapy alone (including the neck) for patients with stage I and II disease; for patients with stage III and IV disease, surgery and radiation therapy is appropriate. The 5-year disease-free survivals are as follows: for patients with stage I cancer, 70% to 80%; for those with stage II, 65% to 75%; for those with stage III, 45% to 50%; and for those with with stage IV, 30%.

Laryngeal cancer accounts for 1.2% of all cancers in the United States, and in 2000, approximately 11,000 new cases will be diagnosed. For patients with either supraglottic laryngeal cancer or glottic laryngeal cancer and smaller tumors, stage I or II, the treatment of choice is radiation therapy, 65 to 70 Gy over 6 to 7 weeks; such radiation therapy results in an excellent cure rate, more than 80% at 5 years. Large tumors, stage III or IV, are best treated with neoadjuvant chemotherapy, cisplatin and 5-FU, followed by radiation therapy, which allows for organ preservation and is preferable to total laryngectomy.

Esophageal Cancer

Esophageal cancer will account for 13,000 new cases and 11,500 deaths in 2000. Esophageal cancer is almost three times more common in men than in women. The risk factors are cigarette smoking, alcohol use, Plummer-Vinson syndrome, achalasia, and tylosis. Barrett esophagus is adenomatous metaplasia of the distal esophagus and is a premalignant lesion that puts patients at risk for adenocarcinoma of the distal esophagus. Patients with gastroesophageal reflux are particularly at risk for Barrett esophagus. Barrett esophagus is associated with a mutant type p53 gene and protein rather than the normal "wild-type."

Symptoms and Signs

The signs and symptoms of esophageal cancer are dysphagia, weight loss, odynophagia, and, rarely, cough. The physical findings fail to demonstrate any specific abnormalities unless patients have obvious organ metastases. Hence, the presence of these symptoms should prompt an esophagography and esophageal endoscopy. After a diagnosis of esophageal cancer has been made, the cancer is clinically staged as shown in Tables 9-2 and 9-3.

Although a decade ago squamous cell carcinoma was the most common histologic subtype of esophageal cancer, today it is adenocarcinoma. The incidence of adenocarcinoma of the distal third of the esophagus at the gastroesophageal junction has increased dramatically in both the United States and Europe. Squamous cell cancer of the esophagus occurs in the proximal two thirds of the esophagus.

Treatment and Prognosis

The treatment of esophageal cancer is either chemoradiotherapy (5-FU, cisplatin, with concurrent radiation therapy) followed by surgery or chemoradiotherapy alone. Although surgery alone may have a role in the treatment in patients with early esophageal cancer, most patients with esophageal cancer have stage IIA–III disease. A randomized trial by the Radiation Therapy Oncology Group (RTOG) conclusively proved the superiority of chemoradiotherapy over radiation therapy alone (1). The 5-year survival was 27% for

Table 9-2 Staging of Esophageal Cancer

Tumor

Tis	Carcinoma in situ
T1	Involvement of lamina propria
T2	Invasion of muscularis
T3	Invasion of adventitia
T4	Invasion of adjacent mediastinal structures

Nodes

N0	No nodal involvement
N1	Nodal metastases

Metastasis

M0	None
M1	Distant metastases

Staging Groups

I	T1, N0, M0
IIA	T2 or T3, N0, M0
IIB	T1 or T2, N1, M0
III	T4, N0, M0
	T1-3, N1, M0
IV	Any T, any N, M1

Table 9-3 Staging Work-up for Esophageal Cancer

Chest radiography
Upper endoscopy
Barium swallow
Computed tomography
  Chest
  Abdomen

---

chemoradiotherapy compared with 0% for radiation therapy alone. Another randomized study trial compared preoperative chemoradiotherapy followed by surgery with surgery alone in 113 patients with adenocarcinoma of the distal esophagus (gastroesophageal junction) (2). The 3-year survival rates were 32% for chemoradiotherapy followed by surgery compared with 6% for surgery alone. Patients with stage IV disease can be palliated with chemotherapy; Taxol, 5-FU, and cisplatin are all active agents.

Lung Cancer

Lung cancer is the leading cause of cancer-related mortality in the United States. Lung cancer is the most common cause of cancer death in American women and in 2000 will account for 75,000 deaths (33,000 more than breast cancer). The number one risk factor for lung cancer is cigarette smoking. Ninety percent of all lung cancers are related to cigarette smoking. Second-hand smoke accounts for about 5000 of the 178,000 new cases of lung cancer anticipated in 2000. Other environmental factors include exposure to arsenic, asbestos, *bis* (chloromethyl) ether, chromium, nickel, radon, and vinyl chloride. Patients who have received external beam radiotherapy for the treatment of Hodgkin's disease or breast cancer are at an increased risk for primary lung cancer. Persons with genetic factors that may contribute to an increased risk of lung cancer include those who either have high levels of 4-debrisoquin hydroxylase or a relative deficiency of glutathione transferase. Because smoking cessation has a significant effect on the incidence of lung cancer, physicians must do all they can to get patients to quit smoking and thus stop the epidemic of lung cancer. Smokers may require counseling, smoking cessation programs, and drugs to treat their nicotine addiction.

Lung cancer begins in a endobronchial stem cell that has the ability to differentiate along multiple lines. Lung cancers are pathologically classified as either small cell or "non–small cell" lung cancer (adenocarcinoma, squamous cell carcinoma, and large cell carcinoma). It is not uncommon to find mixed histologies in a lung cancer such as adenocarcinoma and squamous or small cell and adenocarcinoma. Lung cancer arises from mutational events in the bronchial epithelium, with the cancer occurring as the culmination of 10 to 20 such events. One of the earliest events is allelic loss on the short arm of chromosome 3 that leads to bronchial epithelial hyperplasia. Allelic loss on the short arm of chromosome 9 converts hyperplasia to dysplasia. Mutation of the p53 gene and activation of the K-*ras* oncogene convert dysplasia to carcinoma in situ. A mutation of the p53 gene by compounds in cigarette smoke is a ubiquitous finding in non–small cell lung cancers. In contrast, abnormalities of the short arm of chromosome 3 and the *RB* gene seem to characterize small cell lung cancer (see Chapter 1, p 11).

Symptoms and Signs

The symptoms and signs of lung cancer are dependent on the anatomic location and the extent of disease. Symptoms include cough, hemoptysis, dyspnea, weight loss, fatigue, hoarseness, chest pain, shoulder and arm pain (particularly with superior sulcus tumors [Pancoast tumors]). The physical signs include the presence of consolidative changes ("e to a" with dullness), dullness in the base with diminished breath sounds (pleural effusion), clubbing, superior vena cava syndrome, Horner syndrome (ptosis, mycosis, ipsilateral anhydrosis with apical lung cancer), or signs of metastatic involvement such as lymphadenopathy, hepatomegaly, or neurologic findings. Paraneoplastic syndromes include ectopic adrenocorticotropic hormone syndrome, Eaton-Lambert syndrome, dermatomyositis, and acanthosis nigricans.

To obtain a tissue diagnosis for central lesions, bronchoscopy and biopsy are preferred; for peripheral lesions, fine needle aspirate and cytologic testing is the preferred approach. (Obtaining a tissue diagnosis is discussed in greater detail in Chapter 2.) After a tissue diagnosis has been obtained, the cancer is staged using the staging studies listed in Table 9-4 and illustrated in Figure 9-1. The clinical staging of lung cancer is shown in Table 9-5. Pathologic staging is reserved for patients with clinical stage I lung cancer. Mediastinoscopy is a pathologic staging procedure used in patients with non–small cell lung cancer. It allows the thoracic surgeon to review and inspect the right paratracheal node by making a small incision in the suprasternal notch and inserting a mediastinoscope in the right paratracheal space. A suprasternal mediastinoscopy

Table 9-4 Staging Work-up for Lung Cancer

Chest radiography
Computed tomography
  Chest
  Abdomen

does not allow access to the left paratracheal nodes because of the aortic arch. A left parasternal mediastinotomy allows access to the left-sided mediastinal nodes. Since fluorodeoxyglucose positron emission tomography (FDG PET) came into use, the indications for mediastinoscopy and mediastinotomy are

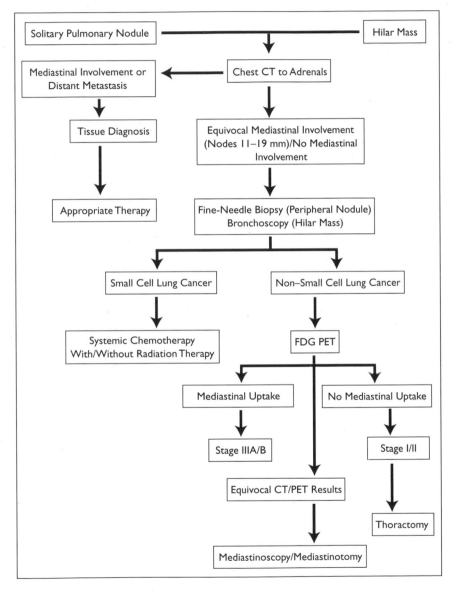

Figure 9-1 Clinical/pathologic staging of lung cancer. CT = computed tomography; PET = positron emission tomography; FDG = fluorodeoxyglucose.

Table 9-5 Staging of Lung Cancer

Primary tumor		Nodal Involvement		Metastases	
Tis	Carcinoma in situ	N0	No regional nodal metastases	M0	No distant metastases
T1	Tumor <3 cm surrounded by lung or visceral pleura	N1	Metastasis to ipsilateral peribronchial or hilar nodes	M1	Distant metastases
T2	Tumor >3 cm or invasion of visceral pleura, or obstructive pneumonitis	N2	Metastases to ipsilateral mediastinal nodes		
T3	Tumor of any size with invasion of chest wall, diaphragm, esophagus, or within 2 cm of carina	N3	Contralateral mediastinal		
T4	Tumor with invasion of mediastinal structures of malignant pleural effusion				

Staging	
Stage 0	Tis, N0, M0
Stage I	T1 or T2, N0, M0
Stage II	T1 or T2, N1, M0
Stage IIIA	T3, N0, N1, M0
Stage IIIB	T1–3, N2, M0
Stage IV	Any T, any N, M1

becoming fewer. Currently, if a patient who has a suspected or proven non–small cell lung cancer has mediastinal lymph nodes less than 1 cm on chest computed tomography (CT) and no uptake in the mediastinum on PET, mediastinoscopy and mediastinotomy do not need to be performed. A thoracotomy should be done. Similarly, if there is obvious mediastinal involvement (mediastinal lymph nodes >2 cm) and uptake in the mediastinum on PET, then mediastinoscopy and mediastinotomy should not be performed. This staging work-up is reserved for patients with equivocal findings on either CT or FDG PET. Pathologic staging is also important as a means of acquiring additional information to help in making treatment decisions. For example, a patient with a right hilar mass and an ipsilateral effusion either may have an operable lung cancer if the effusion is the result of right middle or lower lobe atelectasis or inoperable lung cancer if the effusion is malignant. In this setting, a thoracentesis is mandatory in helping make the appropriate treatment decision.

Treatment and Prognosis

The treatment of lung cancer, both small cell and non–small cell, is dependent on stage. For patients with small cell lung cancer, the backbone of treatment is chemotherapy with simultaneous chemoradiotherapy reserved for patients with "limited stage" (stages I–IIIB) small cell lung cancer. In such patients, chemotherapy consists of cisplatin, 60 mg/m^2 IV on Day 1, and etoposide, 120 mg/m^2 on Days 1, 2, and 3 with simultaneous radiation therapy, 45 Gy/25 fractions to the chest, mediastinum, and bilateral supraclavicular fossae. The chemotherapy is administered for six cycles (18 weeks). If patients achieve a complete response to therapy, it is reasonable to consider prophylactic cranial irradiation to reduce the probability of central nervous system relapse.

The treatment of patients with extensive (stage IV) small cell lung cancer is palliative chemotherapy. The treatment results in patients with limited small cell lung cancer are a 3-year disease-free survival of 30% to 40% and a 5-year disease-free survival of 15% to 20%. The drop off between the third and fifth years is related to late relapses of small cell and the occurrence of new non–small cell primaries. Patients with extensive small cell lung cancer have a median survival of 12 to 14 months.

Patients with "limited" or "extensive" small cell lung cancer who develop progressive disease while receiving treatment with etoposide and cisplatin or who experience relapse after no longer receiving this treatment can be palliated with topotecan. Clinical trials are currently underway exploring the role of topotecan in front-line therapy for small cell lung cancer.

The treatment of patients with non–small lung cancer (NSCLC) depends greatly on the stage of the cancer. Patients with clinical stage I NSCLC are candidates for resection; however, before resection can be considered, these patients should undergo preoperative evaluation including pulmonary function testing to determine whether they are indeed surgical candidates. The pulmonary function testing should include spirometry, measurement of arterial blood gases, diffusion capacity, and, in some instances, quantitative ventilation–perfusion lung scanning. Patients are suitable surgical candidates if their forced expiratory volume in one second (FEV$_1$) is greater than 2.0 L or 70% of predicted, provided that hypercarbia is not present (PCO$_2$ <45 mm Hg, PO$_2$ >70 mm Hg) and that there is no evidence of cor pulmonale. Such patients are assumed to be surgical candidates and should undergo a mediastinoscopy/mediastinotomy to confirm that they are. Patients with an FEV$_1$ of less than 2.0 L require a split quantitative ventilation-perfusion (V/Q) lung scan (Fig. 9-2).

If the mediastinal lymph node biopsies fail to disclose metastatic involvement, lobectomy with a mediastinal dissection (staging) is carried out. Rarely do patients require bilobectomy or pneumonectomy. A wedge or segmental resection is associated with an increased rate of local recurrence and should be avoided unless the patient can not tolerate a lobectomy. The results of surgical therapy in patients with stages IA–IIIA NSCLC are shown in Table 9-6. Patients who present with clinical stage IA or IB NSCLC and who at the time of thoracotomy are found to have metastases to a single mediastinal site (stage IIIA) can be successfully treated with surgical resection (Table 9-6).

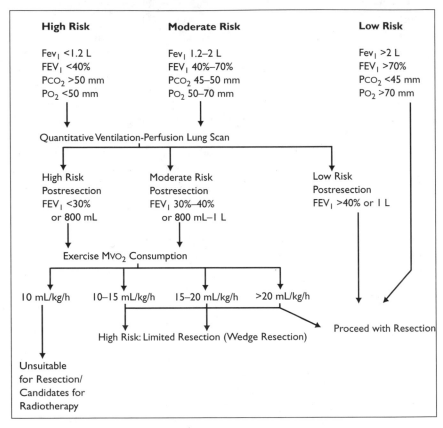

Figure 9-2 Preoperative assessment of clinical stage I non–small cell lung cancer.

Table 9-6 Results of Lobectomy/Pneumonectomy for Stages IA–IIIA NSCLC

Stage	5-year survival (%)
IA	80
IB	60
IIA, IIB	40–50
IIIA	25–30

Case 9-1

An 80-year-old white man was seen in consultation for a second opinion regarding treatment for a newly diagnosed lung cancer. He was in his usual state of relatively good health until January 1999, when he developed a dry, nonproductive cough not associated with fever. A chest radiograph showed a right lower lobe mass that was not found on chest radiography performed in October 1997. Computed tomography of the chest to the level of the adrenals confirmed the presence of a right upper lobe (RUL) mass measuring 3 × 5 cm. The mediastinum appeared normal; the lymph nodes measured less than 1 cm. A bronchoscopy and washings of the RUL were nondiagnostic. A fine-needle aspiration showed an adenocarcinoma. Positron emission tomography showed uptake in the RUL and mediastinum (Fig. 9-3). Despite the PET findings, a right thoracotomy, right lower lobectomy, and mediastinal lymph node dissection were performed. The pathologic findings showed a 5 × 5 cm adenocarcinoma, grade III with metastases to 10 of 18 right mediastinal lymph nodes (stage IIIA).

The patient was advised that no further therapy was indicated because there was no evidence that adjuvant mediastinal irradiation or chemotherapy would in any way alter his disease's course. He was advised that he should be followed closely and that the median survival associated with his stage of NSCLC was 15 to 18 months.

Discussion
This case illustrates the value of PET scan in accurately staging NSCLC. If one had wanted to prove pathologic mediastinal involvement, a mediastinoscopy would have done so. Unlike patients with a single mediastinal lymph node involved, this man does not have a favorable prognosis.

Patients who are not surgical candidates owing to marginal pulmonary function (FEV_1 <1.2 L or postresection FEV_1 <800 mL), cardiovascular disease, or advanced age are best treated with radiation therapy; however, the 5-year survival of patients with stage I and II NSCLC treated with radiotherapy (60–70 Gy) are 20% to 30%.

To date, adjuvant chemotherapy or postoperative radiotherapy does not have a role in the treatment of patients with stage I or II NSCLC. Patients successfully treated for stage I or stage II NSCLC have a 2% to 3% cumulative risk per year of developing a second "new" primary lung cancer. Because of this risk, they should be followed every 3 to 4 months for the first 24 months and every 6 months thereafter. Chest radiography should be done at each visit and CT should be performed annually. Patients with clinical stage IIIA or IIIB NSCLC (clinical mediastinal involvement on CT or PET scan) are best treated with initial chemotherapy (cisplatin, 100 mg/m² intravenously on Days 1 and 29, and vinblastine, 5 mg/m² intravenously weekly) followed

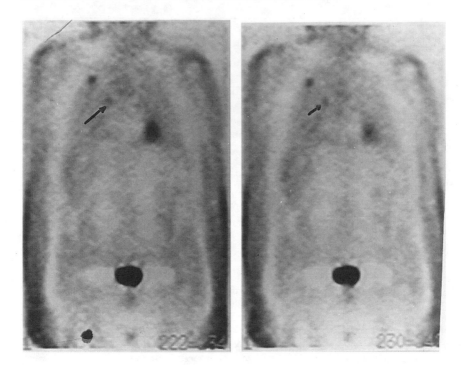

Figure 9-3 A positron emission tomographic (PET) scan of the patient described in Case 9-1. The PET scan shows uptake in the right upper lobe and mediastinum, indicating that the patient had mediastinal involvement and therefore had clinical stage IIIA cancer. This patient had uresectable disease (see text).

by radiation therapy. The median survival of patients treated in such a manner is 14 to 15 months, with a 5-year survival of 20%. Clinical trials are in progress examining other chemotherapeutic regimens, altered radiation therapy fractionation, concurrent chemoradiotherapy approaches, and the addition of antiangiogenesis compounds. Patients should be encouraged to participate in such trials. Patients with stage IIIA or IIIB NSCLC and a poor performance status (i.e., ambulatory less than half of the day [chair- or bed-bound]), are best treated with palliative radiotherapy alone. These patients have an extremely poor prognosis, with a median survival of 9 to 12 months.

Patients with stage IV NSCLC can be palliated with chemotherapy. As the best regimen is as yet unknown, such patients should be encouraged to participate in clinical trials. For those patients with stage IV NSCLC who are ambulatory, without debility from the cancer, and choose not to participate in clinical trials, vinorelbine, etoposide and cisplatin or carboplatin, paclitaxel and carboplatin, taxotere, and gemcitabine are all active agents and can be used to achieve palliation. The median survival of patients with stage IV NSCLC is 8 to 9 months, and the 1-year survival is 35% to 40%.

REFERENCES

1. **Herskovic A, Martz K, al-Sarraf M, et al.** Combined chemotherapy and radiotherapy alone in patients with cancer of the esophagus. N Engl J Med. 1992;326:1593-8.
2. **Walsh TN, Noonan N, Hollywood D, et al.** A comparison of multimodal therapy and surgery for esophageal adenocarcinoma. N Engl J Med. 1996;335:462-7.

Chapter 10

Gastrointestinal Malignancies

Gastric Cancer

Gastric cancer will account for an estimated 22,400 new cases in 2000 and 14,000 deaths will be attributed to it. The incidence of gastric cancer decreased from 1930 to 1970; however, over the past 20 years, the incidence of gastric cancer has remained relatively stable. The incidence of gastric cancer decreases with age and has a male predominance. Multifocal gastric cancer is observed in 20% of all patients. Risk factors include pernicious anemia (although this relationship has been recently questioned) and previous gastric resection.

Symptoms and Signs

The symptoms of gastric cancer are nonspecific and include weight loss, anorexia, early satiety, and pain. Hematemesis occurs in 10% to 15% of all patients with gastric cancer.

The physical findings are referable to the presence of anemia (pallor) and/or metastatic involvement (hepatomegaly, left supraclavicular nodal involvement [Virchow node], and peritoneal implants that are palpable on rectal examination [Blumer shelf]).

The diagnosis of gastric cancer is made on endoscopy with or without double-contrast barium radiography of the stomach. After a diagnosis is made, chest radiography and computed tomography (CT) of the chest, abdomen, and pelvis are undertaken. Computed tomography documents the extent of disease, the presence of liver metastases, or adenopathy in the celiac, retroperitoneal, or porta hepatis regions (see Chapter 3, p 56). The patient is then staged in accordance with the staging classifications shown in Table 10-1. Treatment decisions are then made based on staging.

Treatment and Prognosis

For patients with stages A–B3 gastric cancer (those without nodal metastasis), laparoscopy has emerged as an excellent tool for assessing the extent of disease and its resectability before having the patient undergo a laparotomy. If the patient appears to have "localized disease," the surgeon can perform a laparotomy and subtotal gastrectomy with lymphadenectomy of the paracardial and perigastric lymph nodes (D-1 dissection). More extensive resection of the celiac, left gastric, splenic, and porta hepatic lymph nodes increases the morbidity but does not increase the cure rate. Patients with stages A–B2 gastric cancer, which comprises approximately one third of all patients with gastric cancer, treated surgically have a 5-year survival rate of 20% to 80%, depending on the location of the gastric cancer. Distal tumors carry a worse prognosis. Adjuvant therapy has not been proved to be beneficial and is not required. Patients with stages C1–2 are also treated with surgical resection, but the 5-year survival rate is only 20%; such patients should be encouraged to participate in clinical trials. To date, trials using chemoradiotherapy in this population have not shown a survival advantage. Patients with stage C3 or D gastric cancer are best treated with either palliative resection or bypass surgical procedures that allow them to continue to eat. They may be candidates for clinical trials and should be encouraged to participate. Other options include palliative chemotherapy with 5-fluorouracil (5-FU) with leucovorin or palliative care.

Table 10-1 Staging of Gastric Cancer

Stage	
A	Limited to mucosa
B1	Involvement of gastric wall, no nodal metastases
B2	Involvement of gastric serosa, no nodal metastases
B3	Involvement of adjacent organs, abdominal wall, no nodal metastases
C1	Nodal metastases, limited to gastric wall
C2	Nodal metastases, invasion of entire gastric wall (serosa)
C3	Nodal metastases, invasion of adjacent organs
D	Distant metastases

Pancreatic Cancer

Pancreatic cancer is the fifth leading cause of cancer-related deaths in the United States. In 2000, it is estimated that 28,000 new cases of pancreatic cancer will be diagnosed and 26,500 deaths will result from it. These statistics are staggering to say the least, because more than 90% of patients diagnosed with pancreatic cancer die as a result of the disease. Pancreatic cancer is a highly lethal disease, with a median survival of only 12 weeks and a 5-year survival of only 3%. The problem with pancreatic cancer is that by the time most patients are diagnosed, 80% already have metastatic involvement; for those 20% who appear to have "localized disease," 90% die within the first 24 months from recurrent pancreatic cancer after a curative resection.

The risk factor for pancreatic cancer is cigarette smoking. Unproved risk factors include alcohol, caffeine, and N-nitroso compounds. Most recently, "familial" or hereditary pancreatic cancer has been reported, and in 1988, a familial registry was established. However, the prevailing wisdom is that even if genetics play a role, this would only account for 3% to 5% of all pancreatic cancers.

Symptoms and Signs

The signs and symptoms of pancreatic cancer are anorexia, weight loss, abdominal discomfort or pain, nausea, and jaundice. All of these symptoms are nonspecific or reflect advanced disease and do not lead to an early diagnosis of pancreatic cancer. The pain associated with pancreatic cancer is constant, gnawing, and radiates to the back because of splanchnic plexus invasion. Painless jaundice is a rare symptom in patients with pancreatic cancer, and in more than 90% of cases with this symptom, the jaundice is accompanied by epigastric or back pain. The recent onset of glucose intolerance should alert the physician to the possibility of pancreatic cancer. The presence of any physical findings is usually characteristic of advanced stage pancreatic cancer. Several physical findings indicate advanced stage pancreatic cancer: Courvoisier sign (painless jaundice and a palpable gallbladder), ascites, hepatomegaly, Virchow node (left supraclavicular adenopathy), Trousseau syndrome (migratory thrombophlebitis), Sister Mary Joseph node (periumbilical mass), and a Blumer shelf (peritoneal implants palpable on rectal examination).

In a patient with suspected pancreatic cancer, abdominal/pelvic CT is the imaging procedure of choice. The diagnostic accuracy of CT is high (85%). Moreover, CT accurately predicts the potential resectability of pancreatic cancer; however, one should keep in mind that only 70% of patients with clinically resectable pancreatic cancer truly have surgically resectable disease. Abdominal CT is the procedure of choice in the staging of a known pancreatic cancer or in the work-up of a suspected pancreatic cancer (see Chapter 3, p 57). The staging of patients with pancreatic cancer is shown in Table 10-2.

Treatment and Prognosis

The treatment of patients with resectable pancreatic cancer is a Whipple procedure (pancreaticoduodenectomy). More recently, a pylorus-preserving Whipple procedure has been advocated. The mortality associated with the Whipple procedure is 0% to 15%. The median survival of patients with pancreatic cancer after a Whipple procedure is 12 to 15 months, with a 5-year survival of 20% to 30%. The prognosis is worse for those with nodal involvement. For patients with unresectable pancreatic cancer, surgical palliation still has a role. Choledochojejunostomy or cholecystojejunostomy can relieve jaundice, and gastrojejunostomy can relieve duodenal obstruction. Severe pain may be relieved by alcohol ablation of the celiac plexus.

Most patients with pancreatic cancer have unresectable and/or metastatic disease and should be encouraged to participate in clinical trials so that we may be able to advance the state of the art. Patients with unresectable disease who do not wish to participate in trials can be palliated with chemoradiotherapy (5-FU and 40 Gy). The median survival of patients treated in such a manner is 9.5 months. Patients with metastatic pancreatic cancer who refuse trial participation can be palliated with gemcitabine. The median survival of patients with metastatic pancreatic cancer after treatment with gemcitabine is 5.7 months.

Table 10-2 Staging of Pancreatic Cancer

Tumor

T1a	Limited to pancreas <2 cm
T1b	Limited to pancreas >2 cm
T2	Invasion of duodenum, common bile duct, peripancreatic tissues
T3	Invasion of the stomach, spleen, colon, or blood vessels

Nodes

N0	No nodal involvement
N1	Nodal metastases

Metastasis

M0	None
M1	Distant metastases

Stage Groupings

1	T1–2, N0, M0
2	T3, N0, M0
3	T1–3, N1, M0
4	Any T, any N, M1

Colorectal Cancer

Colorectal cancer is the third leading cause of cancer death and accordingly represents a significant health care problem in the United States. It is estimated that 131,000 persons will be diagnosed in 2000, and approximately 55,000 persons will die of this disease. Colon cancer is more common than rectal cancer. The definition of rectal cancer is any tumor arising below the peritoneal reflection or less than 12 cm from the anal verge. Colon cancer occurs equally in men and women; rectal cancer is slightly more common in men. The mean age of presentation is 60 to 65 years; however, the risk of sporadic colon cancer begins at age 40 years. In contrast, the risk of hereditary colon cancer begins between the ages of 25 and 30 years. The risk factors for colorectal cancer include a diet rich in animal fat (a diet rich in fiber and yellow and green vegetables lowers the risk), adenomatous polyps, inflammatory bowel disease, and genetics (see Chapter 1, p 11). Adenomatous polyposis coli (APC) is a group of hereditary syndromes that includes familial adenomatous polyposis, Gardner syndrome, and Turcot syndrome. In each of these diseases, a germline mutation of the APC gene exists and the colon contains hundreds or thousands of polyps that are microscopically adenomas. In Gardner syndrome, extracolonic features include osteomas of the skull, mandible, and long bones, desmoid tumors, and hypertrophy of the retinal pigment. In Turcot syndrome, the foregoing extracolonic features are associated with malignant brain tumors.

Hereditary nonpolyposis colorectal cancer (HNPCC) exists in two forms: Lynch-1, which is colorectal cancer only, or Lynch-2, hereditary colorectal cancer associated with endometrial, bladder, or hepatobiliary cancer. More recently, the flat adenoma syndrome has been described, which is associated with periampullary carcinoma or hepatoblastoma. Patients with APC or HNPCC should be considered candidates for chemoprevention trials or should be treated with nonsteroidal anti-inflammatory drugs (NSAIDs) such as sulindac or long-term aspirin. Both of these NSAIDs have been shown to induce regression of large bowel polyps and reduce the incidence of colorectal cancer.

Symptoms and Signs

The symptoms of colorectal cancer are varied and include vague abdominal pain, flatulence, and changes in bowel habits with or without rectal bleeding. Right-sided colonic cancer more commonly causes anemia (from chronic blood loss), weakness, vague abdominal pain, and on physical examination a mass may be palpable. Left-sided colonic cancers can cause constipation, abdominal pain, and obstructive symptoms such as nausea and vomiting. Patients with rectal cancer usually present with symptoms of rectal fullness, urgency, changes in bowel movements, bleeding, and tenesmus. The physical findings include pallor, a right lower quadrant mass, and a palpable rectal mass, or the findings may be entirely normal. In patients with metastatic involvement, hepatomegaly may be present or abdominal masses may be palpable. A stool Hemoccult test usually documents the presence of hematochezia. In patients with suspected colorectal cancer, the diagnostic work-up includes colonoscopy and/or barium enema. After a diagnosis of colorectal cancer has been established, a staging work-up with chest radiography and abdominopelvic CT is performed. Patients with rectal cancer should undergo transrectal ultrasonography in addition to the staging studies. The pathologic staging of colon and rectal cancers is shown in Table 10-3.

Treatment and Prognosis

For patients with colon cancer, whether it is right- or left-sided, the treatment is laparotomy and right- or left-sided partial colectomy. For tumors of the sigmoid, treatment is a wide sigmoid resection. The colon cancer is then pathologically staged (Table 10-3). Patients with pathologic stages A and B1 colon cancer have an excellent prognosis, and a 5-year disease-free survival of 75% to 90%; additional therapy is not required. For patients with stage B2 colon cancer, the surgical cure rate is 65% to 75%, and the role of adjuvant chemotherapy is as yet undefined and still under investigation. These patients should be encouraged to participate in clinical trials. Patients with stages C1 and C2 colon cancer should receive adjuvant therapy. Adjuvant chemotherapy with levamisole and 5-FU has been shown in controlled trials to reduce the incidence of colon cancer recurrence by approximately one third and therefore increases the 5-year disease-free survival rate from 47% to 63%. Patients with stage C colon cancer should be urged to participate in the next generation of clinical trials, which are comparing monoclonal antibodies and chemotherapy (leucovorin and 5-FU) to alternative adjuvant chemotherapy regimens. Patients with stages D1 and D2 colon cancer are candidates for palliative chemotherapy with the combination of irinotecan, leucovorin, and 5-FU, which has recently been shown to result in a higher response rate and superior survival compared with leucovorin and 5-FU alone. Newer chemotherapeutic agents include potent inhibitors of thymidylate synthase that are currently in trials, oxaliplatin (di-amino-cyclohexane platinum), and other novel compounds. The median survival of patients with stages D1 and D2 colon cancer is 16 to 20 and 12 to 18 months, respectively. Survival of patients with stage D cancer is greatly influenced by the dominant metastatic site of involvement.

The treatment of rectal cancer is somewhat different than that of colon cancer. Surgical resection, low anterior resection (if the tumor is at least 6 cm

Table 10-3 Staging of Colon and Rectal Cancer

Primary Tumor		Nodal Involvement	
Tis	Carcinoma in situ	N0	No nodal metastases
T1	Tumor confined to mucosa or submucosa	N1	Any nodal involvement
T2	Invasion of muscularis up to serosa	**Metastases**	
		M0	No distant metastases
T3	Invasion through serosa or adjacent organs	M1	Distant metastases
T4	Fistula formation		
T5	Extension beyond adjacent organs		

Staging

Stage	
Stage 0	Tis, N0, M0
Stage A	T1, N0, M0
Stage B1	T2, N0, M0
Stage B2	T3–5, N0, M0
Stage C1	T1 or T2, N1, M0
Stage C2	T3 or T4, N1, M0
Stage D	Any T, any N, M1

from the anal verge) or abdominoperineal resection (if the tumor is 2 to 5 cm from the anal verge), is the treatment of choice for patients with small tumors. Actually, such patients are rare, and true stages A and B1 cancer with adenocarcinoma of the rectum comprise a small minority of rectal cancers.

Obviously, the clinical staging of rectal cancer by sigmoidoscopic examination does not adequately determine the depth of penetration. A good rule to follow is that if the rectal cancer is small (<4 cm), exophytic, and not fixed or tethered, one should proceed with initial surgical resection.

For those patients who truly have stage A or B1 rectal cancer, no further therapy is required, because the 5-year disease-free survival rate is 75% to 82%. For patients with rectal cancers that exceed 4 cm, transrectal ultrasonography should be performed before any treatment is begun to determine the feasibility of initial resection. Transrectal ultrasonography will determine the thickness of the rectal wall and any penetration into the perirectal fat. Most such patients who have transrectal ultrasonography will be found to have at the very least stage B2 disease based on the thickness of the rectal wall and/or involvement of perirectal fat. Nodal involvement cannot be ascertained by ultrasonography; nonetheless, patients with clinical stage B2 disease are candidates for neoadjuvant (preoperative) chemoradiotherapy therapy. The best radiotherapy schedule and the best combination chemotherapy regimen for the neoadjuvant treatment of rectal cancer are as yet unknown. A reasonable approach is to combine preoperative radiotherapy, 30 to 45 Gy over 3 to 4 weeks, with 5-FU, 600 mg/m²/d over 24 hours given by continuous infusion for 5 days, and leucovorin, 25 mg orally every 6 hours for 5 days, or 5-FU, 225 mg/m² continuously over 24 hours by ambulatory infusion pump during the entire course of radiotherapy.

The neoadjuvant chemoradiotherapy leads to a down-staging of the initial rectal cancer and may allow for a low anterior resection. Adjuvant chemotherapy is continued with 5-FU and leucovorin postoperatively. The 5-year disease-free survival for patients with stages B2, C1, and C2 rectal cancer treated with neoadjuvant chemoradiotherapy followed by surgery in turn followed by adjuvant chemotherapy is 67% to 70% at 5 years. The treatment of recurrent rectal cancer is a function of the site or sites of metastatic disease. Local recurrences within the pelvis are manifested by pelvic pain or bleeding and can be palliated with local radiotherapy. Patients with obstructing lesions require diverting colostomy and palliative radiotherapy. The median survival of patients with stage D1 rectal cancer is 18 months. Patients with stage D2 rectal cancer, with metastases to liver or lung, are treated in a manner identical to that used for patients with stage D2 colon cancer (discussed earlier in this section). The median survival of stage D2 patients is 12 to 18 months.

Anal Canal Cancers

Anal canal cancers are quite rare. The risk factors include infection with human immunodeficiency virus and possibly with the human papilloma virus. The symptoms and signs are identical to those of rectal cancer. Obviously, one is more apt to detect a mass in the anal canal on digital rectal examination. Most anal cancers are squamous cell cancer, and treatment is chemoradiotherapy (5-FU, mitomycin-C, and concurrent radiotherapy). The 5-year disease-free survival is 80% to 84%, and surgical resection is not necessary.

Chapter 11

Genitourinary Cancer

Prostate Cancer

Prostate cancer is the most common cancer among American men. An estimated 334,500 men will be diagnosed with prostate cancer in 2000 and approximately 42,000 deaths will result from the disease. The risk of prostate cancer increases yearly in men older than 50 years of age, and unlike other malignancies, there is no peak age or modal distribution. Worldwide, the incidence of prostate cancer is highest in Scandinavian men and lowest among Japanese and Chinese men. The risk factors for prostate cancer include family history (first-degree relative) and race. African-American men have a 9.8% lifetime risk of developing prostate cancer; white men have an 8% lifetime risk. There is no association between prostate cancer and dietary fat, vasectomy, and sexually transmitted disease. Many men with prostate cancer are entirely asymptomatic.

Symptoms, Signs, and Screening

Symptoms related to prostate cancer include bladder outlet obstruction, urinary tract infections, and hematuria; metastatic involvement can provoke bone pain, lower extremity lymphedema, and weakness or paralysis (see Chapter 4, p 73). The prostate examination may reveal an enlarged prostate with a firm area or nodule confined to one lobe or diffuse nodularity of both lobes. With more advanced stage disease, lymphedema, paraparesis, bone pain on percussion of the spine, or lymphadenopathy may be seen.

Currently there is little controversy about the value of screening men for prostate cancer. Prostate cancer is a lethal disease, particularly in men younger than 60 years of age and in African-American men. The median survival of men with metastatic (stage D2) prostate cancer is only 3 years. Screening leads to an earlier diagnosis and the likelihood of a better therapeutic outcome. The current screening recommendations include an annual rectal examination and measurement of serum prostate-specific antigen (PSA) using 4 ng/mL as the upper limit of normal. Measurement of the serum PSA should precede the digital examination. The predictive value of a serum PSA of more than 4 ng/mL and abnormal findings on prostate examination is 50%. Annual screening for prostate cancer in men who have one or more first-degree relatives with prostate cancer or in African-American men should begin at age 40 years. For all other men, screening should begin at age 50 years.

Men with a PSA of more than 4 ng/mL and abnormal findings on prostate examination should undergo prostate ultrasonography and biopsy. If the biopsy fails to disclose prostate cancer, these men are followed up at 6 months and 12 months with a prostate examination and measurement of PSA. If no change is found, they should continue to be followed up annually. If the PSA measurement is the only abnormality or if the prostate examination yields the sole abnormal finding, the current recommendation is to follow such men every 6 months until both tests provide abnormal results, because the positive predictive value of either an abnormal PSA level or abnormal findings on digital examination is less than 30% (Table 11-1).

Almost universally, prostate cancer is graded by the Gleason score. The pathologist examines the prostate biopsy and grades the most well-differentiated regions and the most poorly differentiated regions on a scale of 1 to 5. A score of 1 represents well-differentiated prostate cancer (single, separate, uniform glandular appearance in a close-packed mass), and a score of 5 represents ragged masses of anaplastic carcinoma with little gland formation. The scores in between represent gradations between the extremes. The component scores are added together; the Gleason score thus ranges from 2 to 10. The higher the score, the greater is the likelihood that the prostate cancer has spread beyond the gland and metastasized.

Prostate cancer is staged on the basis of the Gleason score, the PSA level, and the clinical examination (Table 11-2). As shown in Tables 11-3 and 11-4, a correlation between the PSA level and cancer stage exists. The probability of truly localized prostate cancer (stage B or less) when the PSA level is 10 to 20 ng/mL is only 45%. Furthermore, the likelihood of truly localized prostate is only 27% when the PSA level is more than 20 ng/ml. The staging procedures are shown in Table 11-5.

Table 11-1 Screening for Prostate Cancer: Predictive Value and Action Plan

Abnormality	Probability of Prostate Cancer (%)	Action Plan
Abnormal prostate findings on DRE; PSA <4 ng/mL	<30	Follow every 6 months
Normal findings on prostate examination; PSA >4 ng/mL	<30	Follow every 6 months
Abnormal prostate findings on DRE; PSA >4 ng/mL	50	Prostate ultrasonography and biopsy
Abnormal prostate findings on DRE; PSA >4 ng/mL but stable; normal findings of prostate ultrasonography; biopsy showing BPH	<30	Follow with DRE and PSA every 6 months

DRE = digital rectal examination; PSA = prostate-specific antigen; BPH = benign prostatic hyperplasia.

Table 11-2 Staging of Prostate Cancer

Primary Tumor		Nodal Involvement		Metastases	
T1	Clinically occult (T1a <5% of resected specimen, T1b >5% of resected specimen, T1c positive needle biopsy with elevated PSA)	N0	No nodal metastases	M0	No distant metastases
		N1	Single node <2 cm	M1	Distant metastases
		N2	Single node >2 cm <5 cm		
T2	Confined to prostate (T2a <half lobe, T2b >half lobe, T2c both lobes)	N3	Single node >5 cm		
T3	Extracapsular invasion				
T4	Fixed or invasion of adjacent structures				

Staging	
Stage A	T1, N0, M0
Stage A2	T1a, N0, M0
	T1b or T1c, N0, M0
Stage B	T2, N0, M0
Stage C	T3, N0, M0
Stage D1	Any T, N1–3, M0
Stage D2	Any T, any N, M1

Table 11-3 Serum Prostate-Specific Antigen (PSA) Values and its Relation to the Stage of Prostate Cancer

Stage	Serum PSA Value (ng/mL)
A1 & A2 (inapparent tumor, T1)	4–8
B (confined to prostate, T2)	12–40
C (extracapsular extension, T3 or T4)	60–100
D1 or D2 (nodal or visceral involvement)	40–200+

Table 11-4 Relation Between Serum Prostate-Specific Antigen (PSA) and Pathologic Stage in Men with "Localized" Prostate Cancer

Serum PSA (ng/mL)	Patients (n)	Prostate Confined	Capsular Spread	Seminal Vesicles Involved	Seminal Vesicle or Nodal Involvement
0–4	421	325 (77%)	81 (9%)	8 (2%)	8 (2%)
4–10	533	324 (61%)	153 (29%)	19 (3%)	37 (7%)
10–20	311	139 (45%)	94 (30%)	38 (12%)	40 (13%)
>20	251	67 (27%)	63 (25%)	52 (20%)	78 (28%)

Reprinted with permission from Trump DL, Shipley WU, Dilloglugil O, Scardino P. Neoplasms of the prostate. In: Holland JF, Frei E, Bast Jr RO, et al, eds. Cancer Medicine. 4th ed. Baltimore: Williams and Wilkins; 1997.

Table 11-5 Staging Work-up for Prostate Cancer

Chest radiography
Prostate-specific antigen measurement
Transrectal prostate ultrasonography
Computed tomography of the pelvis
Bone scan

Treatment and Prognosis

The treatment of prostate cancer must be individualized and is based on stage and patient age.

Men of any age who have prostate cancer found "incidentally" at the time of transurethral resection of the prostate involving less than 5% of the resected tissue (stage A1) and well differentiated in appearance (Gleason score of 4 or less) should be observed. They should be followed on a twice per year basis with a digital prostate examination and measurement of serum PSA. In contrast, men younger than 65 years and who are otherwise healthy with stage A1 or A2 prostate cancer and a Gleason score of greater than 4 are candidates for radical prostatectomy. Men older than 65 years of age with stage A1 or A2 prostate cancer should be observed; however, many of these men will require treatment such as radiation therapy at some point.

Men younger than 65 years old with stage B prostate cancer, a Gleason score of less than 7, and a serum PSA level of less than 10 ng/mL are candidates for radical prostatectomy (RP). In this setting, RP can lead to a 10-year disease-free survival of 82% to 85%. No randomized studies have compared RP with radiation therapy (external beam or external beam plus interstitial implants). Although some radiation therapy series (1,2) have reported comparable results, the concern is whether radiation therapy can result in comparable 20-year disease-free survivals as reported by some RP series. Clearly, in a patient younger than 65 years old, the 20-year results are the most meaningful. Until evidence shows otherwise, RP is my recommendation for such patients. The complications of RP even when "nerve-sparing procedures" are carried out are impotence and incontinence. Men older than age 65 years with stage B prostate cancer, a Gleason score of less than 7, and a PSA level of less than 10 ng/mL have two treatment options. One option is observation with serum PSA levels measured every 3 months, provided that the PSA level remains stable, and the second option is treatment with initial flutamide and leuprolide followed by external beam and interstitial radiotherapy or conformational radiotherapy with 3-D treatment planing.

Regardless of whether they are younger or older than 65 years of age, men with stage B prostate cancer, a Gleason score of more than 7, and a PSA level of 10 to 20 ng/mL (high probability of extracapsular extension) require therapy. Watching and waiting in this setting is not an option because a Gleason score of more than 7 indicates a biologically aggressive prostate cancer. For men younger than age 65 years, the therapeutic options are RP and initial hormone therapy (bicalutamide [Casodex] or flutamide and leuprolide) followed by radiation therapy (conformational or external beam plus interstitial). For men older than 65 years, initial hormone therapy followed by radiation therapy (conformational or external beam plus interstitial) may be the best option. The 10-year disease-free survival rate in such patients is 45% to 55% (1, 2). Men older than age 65 years with stage B or C prostate cancer, a Gleason score of less than 7, and a PSA level of 10 to 20 ng/mL can initially be observed or given the treatment just described for patients with a Gleason score of more than 7. Men of all ages with "clinical" stage B or C prostate cancer, any Gleason score, and a PSA of more than 30 ng/mL have in all probability either stage D1 or stage D2 disease and are thus incurable. In the absence of symptoms, observation is appropriate. In the presence of symptoms, hormonal therapy is the best initial therapy. At present, continuous hormonal therapy compared with intermittent hormonal therapy is under investigation. The median survival of men with stage D2 prostate cancer treated with hormonal therapy is 3 years. Men with stage D2 hormone refractory prostate cancer can be palliated with mitoxantrone and low-dose prednisone; the median survival of men with hormone refractory prostate cancer is only 10 months.

Table 11-6 summarizes the treatment options for men with prostate cancer.

Table 11-6 Treatment Options for Men with Prostate Cancer

Stage	<Age 65 years	>Age 65 years
A1 incidental, PSA <4 ng/mL	Observation	Observation
A1 incidental or A2, PSA >4 ng/mL	RP	Observation
B, Gleason <7, PSA <10 ng/mL	RP	Observation or hormone Rx and radiotherapy
B, Gleason >7, PSA >10 <20 ng/mL	RP or hormone Rx and radiotherapy	Hormone Rx and radiotherapy
C, Gleason <7, PSA >10 <20 ng/mL	Hormone Rx and radiotherapy	Observation or hormone Rx and radiotherapy
B or C, PSA >30 ng/mL	Hormone Rx	Observation or hormone Rx
D2	Hormone Rx	Hormone Rx
D2 Hormone refractory	Mitoxantrone and prednisone	Mitoxantrone and prednisone

RP = radical prostatectomy; hormone Rx = bicalutamide or flutamide and leuprolide; radiotherapy = external beam + interstitial radiotherapy or conformational radiotherapy.

Urothelial Cancer

Bladder cancer as well as cancers of the ureters and renal pelvis begins as a mucosal abnormality and evolves into a transitional cell cancer as part of a multi-step process. Chromosomal abnormalities reported in bladder include deletions of chromosomes 9 and 17p (p53 gene). Mutations involving both the p53 gene and the *RB* gene have been described. In fact, patients with bladder cancer and p53 mutations have a worse prognosis than do patients with bladder cancer and the "wild-type" p53. At present, it is unknown whether these abnormalities are transforming events that initiate bladder cancer or whether they are the culmination of other antecedent events.

Bladder cancer occurs more commonly in men than women and typically occurs in the fifth and sixth decades of life. Risk factors include cigarette smoking, analgesic abuse, chronic urinary tract inflammation, and aniline dye exposure.

Symptoms and Signs

The symptoms of bladder cancer are painless hematuria, urgency, frequency, and small-volume micturition. Symptoms of metastatic or advanced disease include bone pain, pelvic pain, or lymphedema of the lower extremities. In most cases, patients have no physical findings in the absence of metastasis. In the presence of metastasis, the patient may have bone tenderness, lymphadenopathy, or lymphedema.

Table 11-7 Staging Work-up for Bladder Cancer

Chest radiography
Cystoscopy
Computed tomography of pelvis

Table 11-8 Staging of Bladder and Kidney Cancer

Stage	Bladder	Kidney
0a	Noninvasive papillary cancer	—
0is	Carcinoma in situ (flat tumor)	—
I	Involvement of subepithelial connective tissue	Tumor confined to kidney; no perinephric involvement
II	Muscle invasion, superficial or deep	Tumor involving perinephric fat but confined to Gerota fascia; no invasion of renal vein or renal lymph nodes
III	Invasion of perivesicular fat or prostate, uterus, or vagina	Invasion of renal veins or perirenal lymph nodes
IV	Involvement of pelvis, abdominal wall, lymph nodes, or distant metastases	Distant metastasis

The diagnostic work-up in a patient with suspected bladder cancer begins with cystoscopy. The bladder is inspected and biopsies are performed. If a bladder "polyp" (transitional cell carcinoma of the urinary bladder stage 0) is found, it is removed by transurethral resection (TUR) and fulguration and sent for histopathologic examination. Random biopsies of the bladder are taken to determine the presence or absence of multi-focal disease. In the case of invasive bladder cancer, the cancer is staged after the cystoscopy with chest radiography, abdominal and pelvic computed tomography (CT) with a Foley catheter inserted into the bladder and the bladder filled with air (Table 11-7). The staging system is described in Table 11-8. The pathologic findings usually demonstrate a transitional cell carcinoma with varying degrees of differentiation. Squamous cell carcinoma is a more aggressive form of bladder cancer.

Treatment and Prognosis

After bladder cancer has been staged, treatment decisions are made. Patients with a single bladder "polyp" (stage 0 transitional cell carcinoma of the bladder) are treated with TUR and fulguration and then observed for recurrent disease with cystoscopy biannually.

In the setting of a recurrent bladder "polyp," a repeat TUR and fulguration followed by intravesical therapy with bacille Calmette-Guérin (BCG) is optimal therapy. BCG is a nonspecific form of immunotherapy that may exert its antineoplastic effect through immunologic mechanisms similar to those of a vaccine. Adverse effects of intravesical BCG include fever and urinary frequency and urgency. Indications for intravesical therapy are recurrent bladder polyps, multifocal polyps, diffuse carcinoma in situ, and stage I bladder cancer. Patients with diffuse carcinoma in situ of the urinary bladder recurring after BCG are candidates for cystectomy.

Patients with invasive bladder cancer are treated based on the degree of muscle invasion and the location of the bladder cancer. Patients with stage II bladder cancer (superficial muscle invasion) are candidates for cystectomy. Partial cystectomy is an infrequently performed procedure reserved for patients with bladder cancer confined to the bladder dome and with negative biopsies from elsewhere in the bladder. The 5-year surgical cure rate for stage II bladder cancer is 60% to 80%.

Patients with more invasive bladder cancer stage III or node involvement are candidates for cystectomy followed by adjuvant chemotherapy with methotrexate, vinblastine, doxorubicin, and cisplatin (MVAC). The 5-year disease-free survival rate for this patient subset is 60% to 70%. Neoadjuvant chemotherapy is under investigation. Chemotherapy with radiation therapy is reserved for patients who are not surgical candidates; patients who receive this treatment have a 5-year disease-free survival rate of 30% to 50%.

Patients with stage IV bladder cancer based on nodal involvement are best treated with MVAC chemotherapy. In this subset, there is a finite 5-year survival rate of 35% to 40%. Patients with stage IV bladder cancer on the basis of distant metastasis (M1) are candidates for MVAC therapy; however, in this setting, the median survival is only 13 to 15 months. Patients with stage IV (M1) bladder cancer who are elderly or who have underlying heart disease or renal insufficiency who are not candidates for MVAC can be palliated with paclitaxel, gemcitabine, vinorelbine, or the combination of cisplatin and gemcitabine.

Renal Cell Carcinoma

In 2000, approximately 28,000 cases of renal cell carcinoma will be diagnosed and 11,000 deaths will be associated with the disease. Renal cell carcinoma is more common in men than in women and is a cancer that occurs during the fourth to sixth decades of life. In most patients with renal cell carcinoma, the disease develops sporadically. Risk factors include smoking and obesity. For a small minority of patients, the renal cell carcinoma has a genetic basis; this includes Von Hipple-Lindau disease and a familial form. Deletions of the short arm of chromosome 3 (3p–) are common in both. Renal cell carcinoma arises from the

Table 11-9 Staging Work-up for Renal Cancer

Chest radiography
Intravenous pyelography
Computed tomography
  Abdomen
  Pelvis
Magnetic resonance imaging (optional)
Angiography

---

proximal tubular epithelium and histologically may appear as an adenocarcinoma of clear cells, granular cells, or spindle cells (sarcomatoid variant).

Symptoms and Signs

The symptoms and signs of renal cell cancer include hematuria, anemia, fever, weight loss, flank pain, and polycythemia. The physical findings may reflect the anemia or polycythemia but are usually unremarkable or reflect the presence of metastatic involvement. The diagnostic work-up includes chest radiography, intravenous pyelography, contrast-infused abdominal CT, optional magnetic resonance imaging, and renal angiography (Table 11-9). The staging of renal cell carcinoma is shown in Table 11-8.

Treatment and Prognosis

The treatment of renal cell carcinoma stages I, II, and III is radical nephrectomy. Even in the presence of metastatic involvement, nephrectomy is indicated to palliate hematuria. Patients with metastatic involvement are candidates for interleukin-2 (IL-2), the only FDA-approved drug, either at high dose or low dose. Interleukin-2 results in a 14% response rate, with a 5% complete response rate, and the median duration of response is 20 months. The toxicities of IL-2 include chills, fever, myalgias, skin erythema, and hypotension from a capillary leak syndrome. The best responses are observed in patients with lung metastases. Patients with bone and liver involvement tend not to respond to IL-2.

Testis Cancer

In 2000, testis cancer will develop in 7200 young men between the ages of 15 and 35 years. Testis cancer is rare in African-American men and most commonly occurs in white men.

Most testicular cancers are germ cell origin, and 90% of all germ cell tumors arise in the testis. Only 10% arise in extragonadal sites. Risk factors include previous testis cancer, cryptorchidism, Klinefelter syndrome, and Down syndrome.

Symptoms and Signs

The signs and symptoms of testis cancer are a painless scrotal mass with an associated hydrocele in 20% of patients. Other symptoms include back pain usually relieved with heat or hot baths (retroperitoneal adenopathy) or gynecomastia. The physical findings include a testicular mass, abdominal masses or fullness, supraclavicular adenopathy, or hepatomegaly. If a testicular mass is palpated, it should be considered a malignancy until proved otherwise.

Testicular ultrasonography can certainly confirm the presence of a mass; however, ultrasonongraphy cannot differentiate a benign tumor from a malignant one. Hence the diagnostic and therapeutic approach is to draw a serum β-human chorionic gonadotropin (β-HCG) and α-fetoprotein (AFP) and refer the patient to a urologist for a high inguinal orchiectomy.

After a diagnosis of testis cancer has been made, the cancer is staged with chest radiography and CT of the chest, abdomen, and pelvis (Table 11-10). The staging of testis cancer is shown in Table 11-11.

Treatment and Prognosis

Testis cancer is classified histologically into seminoma and nonseminomatous tumors (embryonal carcinoma, choriocarcinoma, teratoma, and endodermal

Table 11-10 Staging Work-up for Testis Cancer

Chest radiography
Computed tomography of abdomen and pelvis
Position emission tomography (optional)

Table 11-11 Staging System for Testis Cancer

Stage	
I	Cancer confined to testis
II	Nodal involvement
IIA	N1, N2a: Fewer than six lymph nodes, no node >2 cm
IIB	N2b: Six or more lymph nodes or any node >2 cm
IIC	N3: Bulky nodal disease; lymph node >5 cm
III	Supradiaphragmatic nodal involvement
IV	Metastases to lung, liver, bone

sinus tumor [yolk sac tumors]). The treatment of seminoma is radiation therapy. For patients with clinical stage I disease, radiation therapy is delivered to a portal that includes the para-aortic lymph nodes and the ipsilateral hemipelvis including the inguinal scar to a dose of 25 to 30 Gy. The toxicities of radiation therapy include mild nausea, vomiting, and diarrhea. Patients with stage II seminoma are treated with radiation therapy that is delivered to a widened portal that includes the ipsilateral pelvis, para-aortic region, mediastinum, and supraclavicular region to a dose of 25 to 30 Gy. Patients with stage III or IV seminoma are treated with chemotherapy (cisplatin, 20 mg/m^2 intravenously on Days 1 through 5; etoposide, 100 mg/m^2 intravenously on Days 1 through 5, every 21 days; bleomycin, 30 IU/wk intravenously [i.e., on Days 1, 8, 15, 22, and so on] [PEB]). The cure rates for seminoma stages I through III are in excess of 95%.

Patients with clinical stage I or II (N1 or N2) nonseminomatous testis cancer are candidates for retroperitoneal lymphadenectomy. The lymphadenectomy should be unilateral and nerve sparing, to help maintain ejaculatory function. Patients with pathologic stage I testis cancer (no nodal involvement at lymphadenectomy) require no further therapy, because the 5-year disease-free survival rate is greater than 98%. After lymphadenectomy, patients with pathologic stage II (N1 or N2) nonseminomatous testis cancer can either receive two courses of adjuvant chemotherapy with PEB or be followed and treated with chemotherapy at relapse. Although nerve sparing unilateral lymphadenectomy helps maintain ejaculatory function, it is far from uniform in its results. Some men will experience retrograde ejaculation and hence be unable to father children. This issue may be particularly relevant in unmarried men in their twenties and thirties. In an attempt to avoid the this potential result of lymphadenectomy in young men with clinical stage II nonseminomatous testis cancer, a reasonable alternative to lymphadenectomy is adjuvant chemotherapy with PEB for 9 weeks. The potential sterility from PEB is quite low and PEB has no effect on ejaculation (see Case 11-1). With either treatment, the 5-year disease-free survival rate is 96%.

Case 11-1

A 24-year-old white man sought medical attention from a urologist after noticing a painless lump in the left testis. The urologist ordered measurement of serum α-fetoprotein and β-HCG and chest radiography, and advised a left high inguinal orchiectomy. The pathologic findings of the left testis included an embryonal cell carcinoma with few seminomatous elements. The findings of the chest CT were normal. Abdominal/pelvic CT showed a single enlarged 1.5-cm left para-aortic lymph node. Positron emission tomography showed uptake in the left para-aortic

Continued.

Case 11-1—cont'd

region that corresponded to the 1.5-cm lymph node apparent on the abdominal CT scan.

His treatment options were unilateral nerve-sparing lymphadenectomy and observation or chemotherapy with PEB for 9 weeks. This young man was recently engaged to be married and wanted the ability to father children. After much discussion, the treatment pathway chosen was chemotherapy with PEB, which was administered January through March 1996. He was married in September 1997. In January 1999, his wife delivered a healthy 7-lb baby boy. The patient has been without recurrent disease for the past 39 months.

Table 11-12 Criteria for Good-risk and Poor-risk Nonseminomatous Testis Cancer

Good Risk	Poor Risk
AFP <10,000 ng/mL	AFP >10,000 ng/mL
β-HCG <50,000 IU/L	β-HCG >50,000 IU/L
LDH <10 times normal	LDH >10 times normal
Pulmonary metastases	Hepatic, bone, or visceral metastases other than lung

AFP = α-fetoprotein; HCG = human chorionic gonadotropin; LDH = lactate dehydrogenase.

Patients with stage III nonseminomatous testis cancer should have prognostic factors considered and segregated on the basis of risk, good or poor, as shown in Table 11-12, because the cure is a function of risk. In good-risk patients, four courses of PEB should be administered, and the resultant 5-year disease-free survival rate is more than 90%. In poor-risk patients, the PEB regimen is used for four cycles but the resultant 5-year disease-free survival rate is less than 50%. In poor-risk patients, alternative chemotherapy regimens appear to be no better than PEB. If residual masses persist after PEB therapy, surgical resection should be considered. If persistent disease is documented after resection, an ifosfamide-based regimen should be employed (etoposide, ifosfamide, and cisplatin [VIP]). In the event of residual or recurrent disease, high-dose chemotherapy and autologous bone marrow transplantation is a consideration.

Gynecologic Cancer

Ovarian Cancer

In 2000, ovarian cancer will be diagnosed in 27,000 women and will account for 14,000 deaths. Ovarian cancer is a disease that most often afflicts post-

Table 11-13 Staging of Ovarian Cancer

Stage	
IA	Confined to one ovary
IB	Confined to both ovaries
IC	Extracapsular extension or positive cytologic test results
IIA	Involvement of the uterus or fallopian tubes
IIB	Involvement of other parametrial tissues
IIC	As above with positive cytologic test results
IIIA	Involvement of the true pelvis with abdominal metastases
IIIB	Abdominal metastases <2 cm
IIIC	Abdominal metastases >2 cm
IV	Visceral metastases

menopausal women (ages 50 to 75 years). Although ovarian cancer is more common in white women than in African-American women, the highest incidence is in Jewish women of Eastern European ancestry (Ashkenazi Jews); this may be related to the relatively high frequency of *BRCA1* mutations in Ashkenazi Jewish women. The cause of epithelial ovarian cancer is unknown as are risk factors other than genetic factors. Hereditary cancer syndromes that predispose to ovarian cancer include hereditary nonpolyposis colorectal cancer (HNPCC), Lynch II, and *BRCA1* and *BRCA2* mutations. Most ovarian cancers are epithelial and classified based on the degree of differentiation. Stromal and germ cell tumors account for fewer than 10% of all ovarian tumors.

Symptoms and Signs

Ovarian cancer is an insidious disease and may produce no symptoms or symptoms such as abdominal distention, abdominal cramps, or diarrhea. It is with such protean symptoms that patients are initially diagnosed with dyspepsia or irritable bowel disease. With more advanced disease, patients may have symptoms of abdominal bloating or swelling, an increase in abdominal girth, frequency, tenesmus, or respiratory distress. The physical finding in early-stage ovarian cancer is a pelvic mass that is usually discovered by chance on a routine pelvic examination. In patients with more advanced disease, there may be ascites, right-sided pleural effusion (Meigs syndrome), complex pelvic masses, or an omental mass.

No screening tests for ovarian cancer exist, and screening "normal" women with ultrasonography or CA-125 is ill advised. However, screening of high-risk patients is advised; high-risk patients include women with known *BRCA1* and *BRCA2* mutations, a family history of HNPCC, or a family history of breast cancer in a first-degree relative younger than age 40

Table 11-14 Staging Work-up for Ovarian and Endometrial Cancer

Chest radiography
Endovaginal ultrasonography
Computed tomography
  Abdomen
  Pelvis
Barium enema

Table 11-15 Treatment of Ovarian Cancer and Resultant 5-year Disease-Free Survival (DFS)

Stage	Grade	Treatment	5-year DFS (%)
IA/B	I–II	TAH, BSO, and omentectomy	90–98
IC, II	II–IV	TAH, BSO, omentectomy, and PT	70–80
IIIA/B	Any	TAH, BSO, omentectomy, and PT	45
IIIC	Any	TAH, BSO, omentectomy, and PT	<10
IV	Any	TAH, BSO, omentectomy, and PT	<3

TAH = total abdominal hysterectomy; BSO = bilateral salpingo-oophorectomy; PT = cisplatin or carboplatin and paclitaxel.

years. In these high-risk patients, biannual transvaginal ultrasonography should be performed and CA-125 should be measured.

To diagnose ovarian cancer, an exploratory laparotomy is necessary. A complete history and physical examination should be performed and a serum CA-125 should be measured. In women younger than age 30 years with a pelvic mass, a serum β-HCG and AFP should be measured, because a germ cell tumor of the ovary is likely. The staging of ovarian cancer is based on the pathologic findings. The staging of ovarian cancer is shown in Table 11-13, and the staging work-up is shown in Table 11-14.

Treatment and Prognosis

The treatment of ovarian cancer is surgical and should be performed by a gynecologic oncologist. The surgical procedure usually is an exploratory laparotomy with a careful inspection of the entire abdominal cavity and its contents. Ascites fluid is sent for cytologic testing, and in the absence of ascites, peritoneal washings for cytologic examination are obtained. The undersurface of the diaphragm, the paracolic gutters, and the omentum are inspected, and biopsy of any suspicious lesions is performed. The para-aortic nodes are inspected and sampled, after which a total abdominal hysterectomy, bilateral salpingo-oophorectomy, and omentectomy are performed. For women of child-bearing age with stage IA or B ovarian cancer, it may be possible to perform a unilateral salpingo-oophorectomy and omentectomy. In women with stage IIIC or even stage IV disease, an experienced gynecologic oncologist should carry out maximum surgical debulking. This is done even if an exploratory laparotomy has already been done and a diagnosis has been made but the patient still has residual ovarian cancer.

Patients with stage IA or IB ovarian cancer and a histologic grade I or II require no further therapy other than surgery. The 5-year disease-free survival rate for this patient subset is 90% to 98% (Table 11-15). Patients with stage IC or stage II ovarian cancer are candidates for adjuvant chemotherapy with cisplatin or carboplatin in combination with paclitaxel (Taxol). The cisplatin/carboplatin and paclitaxel regimen is dosed as follows: cisplatin is administered at a dose of 75 mg/m^2 or carboplatin is dosed at an area under the curve (AUC) of 5 mg/mL/min; paclitaxel is administered at 135 mg/m^2 every 21 days for six courses. The resultant 5-year disease-free survival rate is 70% to 80% (see Table 11-15). Patients with stage IIIA/B ovarian cancer should be treated with the cisplatin/carboplatin and paclitaxel regimen for a minimum of eight cycles. These patients are potentially curable with this chemotherapy program, and the resultant 5-year disease-free survival rate is 45% (see Table 11-15). Patients with stage IIIC and IV ovarian cancer can be palliated with chemotherapy, cisplatin/carboplatin and paclitaxel; the median survival is 18 to 24 months. Toxicities associated with cisplatin/carboplatin and paclitaxel include myelosuppresion, myalgias, peripheral neuropathy, renal insufficiency and hearing loss.

Patients with advanced ovarian cancer who relapse after treatment with cisplatin/carboplatin and paclitaxel chemotherapy can be further palliated with topotecan 1.5 mg/m^2/d for 5 days, or liposomal doxorubicin (Doxil), vinorelbine, or external beam radiotherapy.

Case 11-2

In February 1991, a 42-year-old, otherwise healthy white woman consulted her internist after finding a lump in her left breast. The internist noted a dominant mass that was located in the lateral lower quadrant of the left breast at the 5 o'clock position and that measured 1.5 cm. The patient related that her mother had developed breast cancer at age 40 years and had died at age 43 years. The patient also had a maternal aunt who developed breast cancer at age 47 years. The patient was referred to a surgeon and had mammography and ultrasonography of the left breast, which were nondiagnostic. An excisional biopsy showed an infiltrating ductal breast cancer that was 1.2 cm in size. The margins were uninvolved. A left axillary lymph node sampling showed 0 of 19 lymph nodes involved. The patient was given radiation therapy to the left breast and was treated with adjuvant tamoxifen, 10 mg orally twice daily. She was advised to have genetic linkage testing for breast

Continued.

Case 11-2—cont'd

cancer (formal genetic testing was in its infancy at that time) because the family history was suggestive of genetic breast cancer. She declined. She was also advised to undergo biannual ultrasonography of her ovaries and biannual measuremnt of CA-125. She did well until August 1995, when her CA-125 became elevated, increasing from a baseline of 26–30 U/µL to 75 U/µL. She was referred to a gynecologic oncologist, who performed a pelvic examination, transvaginal ultrasonography, and CT that were all "normal." On the gynecologic oncologist's recommendation, CA-125 testing was repeated 3 months later and was found to have increased to 310 U/µL. A repeat pelvic examination was unremarkable; however, transvaginal ultrasonography now revealed a pelvic mass, and exploratory laparotomy and surgical debulking were performed. The findings disclosed stage IIIC ovarian cancer. The residual disease after surgical debulking was less than 2 cm.

The patient was treated with systemic chemotherapy that consisted of paclitaxel given over 24 hours and cisplatin for eight cycles. At that time she was believed to be disease free. She declined a second-look laparotomy but consented to a laparoscopy that failed to disclose any abnormalities. She did well for 18 months (June 1997 through January 1998), but then developed recurrent disease based on a rising CA-125 level. She has been receiving chemotherapy ever since.

Discussion

This woman had a family history that should make a physician suspicious about genetic breast cancer. Although it was not proved that she had a *BRCA1* mutation, in this case the physician should have assumed that she did and should have screened for ovarian cancer. The error made in this woman's situation was the failure to perform a laparoscopy/laparotomy in August 1995, at the first elevation of the CA-125 level. Had aggressive intervention been undertaken at that time, she might be disease-free today. *In the setting of a woman in whom genetic breast cancer is suspected, it must be assumed that an elevated CA-125 level is reflective of ovarian cancer until proven otherwise.*

Endometrial Cancer

In 2000, adenocarcinoma of the endometrium will be diagnosed in 34,900 women and will claim 5900 lives, making it the seventh leading cause of cancer-related death in women.

Adenocarcinoma of the endometrium is a disease primarily of postmenopausal women, although a full 25% of all patients with endometrial cancer are premenopausal. Risk factors for endometrial cancer include unopposed estrogens, obesity, nulliparity, and the use of tamoxifen for more than 5 years.

Symptoms and Signs

The symptoms and signs of endometrial cancer are abnormal vaginal discharge or vaginal bleeding. In fact, among the general population, 15% of all postmenopausal women who present with the symptom of vaginal bleeding are ultimately found to have endometrial cancer. Other symptoms include pelvic pressure or bladder pressure. The physical findings are uterine enlargement or a pelvic mass. Vaginal bleeding in a postmenopausal woman or heavy and irregular bleeding in a premenopausal woman should prompt a dilation and curettage. After a diagnosis of endometrial cancer has been made, the staging work-up is done as shown in Table 11-14.

The next step is referral to a gynecologic oncologist. The surgical approach is an exploratory of the abdominal cavity with a careful inspection of the peritoneal cavity, fluid samples for cytologic testing, intraperitoneal washings, biopsy of any suspicious lesions, and biopsy of any suspicious pelvic or para-aortic lymph nodes. Once this is completed, the fallopian tubes are clipped or ligated shut and extrafascial hysterectomy and bilateral salpingo-oophorectomy are performed. The cancer is ultimately staged based on the pathologic findings as shown in Table 11-16.

Treatment and Prognosis

The treatment of endometrial cancer is surgery and radiation therapy. The stage, grade, and depth of myometrial penetration determine the extent of radiotherapy. Risk groups have been defined for recurrent disease (Table 11-17).

Table 11-16 Staging of Endometrial Cancer

Stage	
IA	Confined to the endometrium
IB	Involvement of less than one half of the myometrium
IC	Involvement of more than one half of the myometrium
IIA	Extension to the endocervix
IIB	Extension into cervical stroma
IIIA	Extension into serosa and/or positive cytologic test results
IIIB	Extension into vagina
IIIC	Lymph nodal involvement, pelvic or para-aortic
IVA	Bladder or bowel invasion
IVB	Visceral metastases

Table 11-17 Risk of Recurrent Endometrial Cancer as a Function of Stage and Grade

Risk	Probability of Recurrence (%)
Low risk	
Stage IA, grade I	I
Stage IB, grade I or II, <1/3 myometrial invasion	6
Intermediate risk	
Stage IA and B, grade 3	15
Stage IC, all grades	15
Stage IIA and B	30
High risk	
Stage III, IV, clear cell or papillary serous histologic findings	50–80

Depending on the risk group, the following treatment recommendations with regard to radiation therapy are prudent:

1. Stage IA or IB, Grade I or II: No adjunctive radiotherapy.
2. Stage IA or B, Grade 3, and Stage IC: Radiation therapy to the whole pelvis, 45 to 50 Gy with vaginal radiotherapy (intracavitary, high or low dose rate).
3. Stage IIA or B: Postoperative radiotherapy to the whole pelvis, 45 to 50 Gy, and intracavitary vaginal radiotherapy with a vaginal cylinder to a total dose of the vaginal surface of 80 to 90 Gy.
4. Stage III: Women with stage III endometrial cancer are at extremely high risk for intra-abdominal involvement and accordingly aggressive radiotherapy is required. These patients require whole abdominal radiotherapy, 20 Gy in 100-cGy fractions followed by an additional 20 Gy to the pelvis, and intracavity vaginal radiotherapy. Women with nodal involvement require an extension of the pelvic portal to include the para-arotic lymph nodes.
5. Stage IV: Women with stage IVA disease receive treatment similar to that given to stage III patients; however, the total pelvic dose is 50 Gy.

Women who are poor surgical risks can be treated with primary radiotherapy, which includes both intracavitary intrauterine radiotherapy and external beam radiotherapy. Primary radiotherapy results are comparable to those for surgery and radiotherapy. Table 11-18 summarizes the treatment outcomes for women with endometrial cancer stages I–IVA if treated with surgery and radiotherapy or primary radiotherapy.

Women with stage IVB endometrial cancer (visceral metastasis) can be palliated through the judicious use of either hormonal therapy or chemotherapy.

Table 11-18 Five-year Disease-Free Survival (DFS) Rate for Women with Endometrial Cancer

Stage	Surgical Treatment	5-year DFS	
		Surgery and Radiotherapy (%)	Primary Radiotherapy (%)
IA, grade I	TAH and BSO	94	87
IA, IB, grade I or II	TAH and BSO	92	87
IA, IB, Grade 3, or IC	TAH, BSO, and RT	80	78
II	TAH, BSO, and RT	70–80	68
IIIA and B	TAH, BSO, and RT	60–70	60
IIIC and IVA	TAH, BSO, and RT	45–50	45–50

TAH = total abdominal hysterectomy; BSO = bilateral salpingo-oophorectomy; RT = radiotherapy.

In women with well-differentiated endometrial cancer and expression of either estrogen or progesterone receptors, one should administer a trial of megestrol acetate, 40 to 320 mg daily, or medroxyprogesterone, 400 to 1000 mg intramuscularly weekly for 8 to 10 weeks followed by same dose monthly. The median survival is 1 year; the 4-year survival rate is 15%. Tamoxifen has been used in women with endometrial cancer and is an active drug but appears to be no more effective than progestational agents.

Chemotherapeutic drugs and combinations should be used in women with stage IVB poorly differentiated endometrial cancer, those patients with stage IVB cancer who have papillary or serous histologic findings, and women who do not respond to progestational agents. If a clinical trial is available, such patients should be encouraged to participate. In patients with papillary or serous histologic findings and visceral involvement (lungs, liver, bone), the combination of cisplatin and paclitaxel, as in ovarian cancer, should be used. For women with all other histologic findings and with nonvisceral metastases, it is best to use single-agent cisplatin, paclitaxel, or doxorubicin. If visceral involvement is present, the combination of doxorubicin and cisplatin should be used. Women with hormone refractory endometrial cancer have a life expectancy of 1 year.

REFERENCES

1. **Bagshaw MA, Kaplan ID, Cox RC.** Prostate cancer: radiation therapy for localized disease. Cancer. 1993;71:939-52.
2. **Bagshaw MA, Cox RS, Hancock SL.** Control of prostate cancer with radiotherapy: long-term results. J Urol. 1994;152:1781-5.

Chapter 12

Breast Cancer

Breast cancer is the most common malignancy in women. In 2000, 181,600 women will be diagnosed with breast cancer and approximately 43,000 will die of this disease. Mortality associated with breast cancer has decreased by 2% to 3% since 1997. This decline in mortality is the result of earlier diagnosis through the use of screening mammography and adjuvant therapies. We are reaping the benefits today from the adjuvant clinical trials started in the 1970s. Clearly, as adjunctive therapies improve through the current generation of trials, the number of deaths resulting from breast cancer will continue to fall.

Risk factors for breast cancer include genetic mutations of *BRCA1* and *BRCA2*, Li-Fraumeni syndrome (mutant p53 protein), Cowden disease, proliferative breast disease, a family history, early menarche, nulliparity, obesity, increased dietary fat intake, and previous radiation exposure. Early menarche and nulliparity create risk by continuous and unopposed (by pregnancy) cyclic estrogen and progesterone synthesis. Although a debate has raged over the risk created by weight and dietary fat, the consensus at this time is that they do increase the risk of breast cancer. One hypothesis is that women with high body fat content may have greater peripheral aromatase enzymatic activity and presumably have higher circulating estradiol levels than their nonobese counterparts. Proliferative breast disease, ductal hyperplasia, atypical ductal hyperplasia, and lobular carcinoma in situ all increase breast cancer risk. In my opinion, women with atypical ductal hyperplasia have a premalignant process, as the risk of developing breast cancer is increased fivefold. The fact is that 1.5% of women with atypical ductal hyperplasia develop breast cancer yearly, and the risk is cumulative—that is, 15% at 10 years, 30% at 20 years, and so on. Lobular carcinoma in situ is not actually a form of breast cancer. Rather, it is a premalignant lesion and serves as a sentinel for women whose risk of developing a *ductal breast cancer is increased eightfold*. A better term for this process is *lobular neoplasia*. Any family history increases the risk 1.7-fold; a mother or a sister with a history of breast cancer increases the risk fourfold. Although familial breast cancer only accounts for 5% of all breast cancer diagnosed, genetic mutations of *BRCA1* and *BRCA2* place women at risk (see Chapter 1, p 14). The lifetime risk of breast cancer for a woman with a *BRCA1* mutation is 65% to 85%; for those with a *BRCA2* mutation, the lifetime risk is 35% to 50%. The Li-Fraumeni syndrome and Cowden disease also increase the risk of breast cancer (see Chapter 1, p 12). Women with previous exposure to radiation, particularly women treated with mantle radiation therapy for Hodgkin disease, are at high risk for breast cancer, usually after a 10-year latency period. Because many of these women with Hodgkin disease were in their late teens and early twenties when they received radiation therapy, they represent a group of women younger than age 35 years who are at risk for breast cancer.

Despite the controversy regarding the age at which to start screening mammography, mammography as a screening tool is clearly beneficial and can reduce mortality from breast cancer. Within the United States, the stage distribution of breast cancer has shifted as a result of mammography: Many more women are now diagnosed with stage I breast cancer than were a decade earlier. Although mammography is not foolproof, it is the best screening tool available to date. The current recommendations for women who are not considered to be at high risk (e.g., no history to suggest familial breast cancer, no history of previous radiotherapy to the chest region) are that screening mammography start at age 40 years and be performed every 1 to 2 years thereafter. For women who are considered to be at high risk, screening with mammography should begin at age 30 years and be performed every 1 to 2 years.

Signs, Symptoms, and Diagnostic Approach

Women with breast cancer may present with a complaint of a "lump" (dominant lump) within the breast (65% to 70%), breast pain (5%), skin or nipple retraction (5%), nipple discharge (2%), or nipple curling or erosion (1%), or they may be entirely asymptomatic. A dominant lump is defined as a palpable mass within the breast that is distinct from the otherwise lumpy consistency of the breast tissue. The mass may be firm (not necessarily rock-hard), movable (not necessarily fixed), or even painful (the presence of pain does not rule in or rule out breast cancer). A mammographic abnormality may have been found by the woman and that may be what has prompted her visit to the physician. In 14% to 21% of the visits, the physician discovers a dominant lump in an otherwise asymptomatic woman.

The diagnostic approach to women with a dominant lump is shown in Figure 12-1. As shown in this algorithm, the diagnostic approach differs slightly in women who are premenopausal (arbitrarily defined as younger than 49 years) compared with postmenopausal women. Obviously, the approach is different if a mammographically identified abnormality without a palpable lump is found. In women with a mammographically identified abnormality, the diagnostic approach is to perform either a stereotactic fine-needle biopsy or a needle localization and excisional biopsy with mammography of the excised breast specimen (to be certain that the area in question has been removed for histopathologic examination).

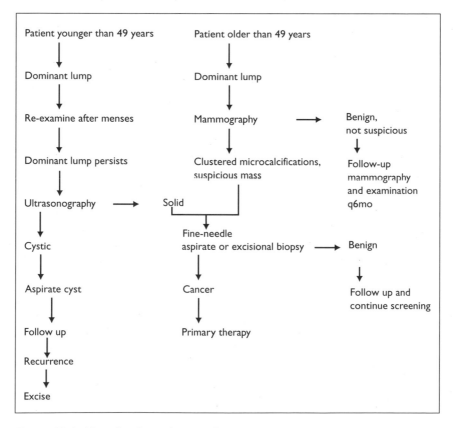

Figure 12-1 Algorithm for evaluation of a breast lump.

Once a diagnosis of breast cancer has been made, additional testing above and beyond the routine pathologic evaluation is necessary. Today, immunohistochemical stains for estrogen and progesterone receptors are mandatory, as is testing for *Her-2/neu* overexpression. Additional tests such as S-phase analysis and ploidy are done in most hospitals but seldom influence treatment decisions.

Ductal Carcinoma In Situ/Lobular Carcinoma In Situ Treatment and Prognosis

Breast cancer may be either invasive or not invasive. Forms of breast cancer that are not invasive include lobular carcinoma in situ (LCIS) and ductal carcinoma in situ (DCIS). Lobular carcinoma in situ, as mentioned earlier, is not actually a form of breast cancer; the better term is *lobular neoplasia*. Lobular neoplasia is a marker that identifies women at risk for developing invasive breast cancer. Lobular carcinoma in situ usually is discovered as an incidental finding on biopsy. It is not a mammographic abnormality. It most commonly occurs in premenopausal women (peak age of onset 45 years). Lobular carcinoma in situ can be multifocal and bilateral and is most often associated with infiltrating lobular carcinoma or tubular histologies. Women with LCIS need to be followed closely. Mastectomy is unnecessary. Women with LCIS are candidates for the current generation of chemoprevention trials (tamoxifen versus raloxifene), or if they decline participation, tamoxifen for a 5-year period with close observation. *Ductal carcinoma in situ* is a term that describes all breast epithelial carcinoma in situ that does not conform in histologic appearance to LCIS. Women with DCIS may present with either a palpable mass or an occult mammographic abnormality that in most cases is either microcalcifications alone or a tissue density with microcalcifications. The peak age of DCIS is 51 to 59 years. Women diagnosed with DCIS have stage 0 breast cancer (Table 12-1). If they are using hormone replacement therapy, it should be discontinued. The treatment approach in such women is to treat the DCIS and minimize the risk of invasive breast cancer. The treatment for DCIS is either a simple mastectomy or lumpectomy and radiation therapy (breast conservation therapy). Decisions governing who is best suited for breast conservation and who is a candidate for simple mastectomy are based on the nuclear grade of DCIS, the presence or absence of a positive margin, the multicentricity of DCIS, and the presence of central necrosis (comedo features). The biologic differences in DCIS based on grade are shown in Table 12-2.

Based on the histologic grade, the frequency of relapse in patients with low-grade DCIS is 2% at 5 years and 15% at 10 years; in contrast, the fre-

Table 12-1 Staging of Breast Cancer

Primary Tumor		Nodal Involvement	
Tis	Ductal carcinoma in situ	N0	No palpable ipsilateral axillary nodes
T1	Tumor <2 cm (T1a < 5 mm, T1b 5–9 mm, T1c >10 mm)	N1	Movable ipsilateral axillary lymph nodes
T2	Tumor >2 cm <5 cm	N1a	No clinical metastases
T3	Tumor >5 cm in size	N1b	Clinical metastases
T4	Tumor of any size with extension to chest wall	N2	Fixed and matted axillary nodes
		N3	Supraclavicular or infraclavicular nodes
		Metastases	
		M0	No distant metastases
		M1	Distant metastases

Staging	
Stage 0	Tis, N0, M0
Stage I	T1, N0, N1a, M0
Stage II	T0 or T1, N1b, M0
	T2, N1a, N1b, M0
Stage IIIA	T3, N0, N1 or N2, M0
Stage IIIA	Inflammatory carcinoma
Stage IV	T4, or N3, or M1

Table 12-2 Biologic Differences in Ductal Carcinoma In Situ Based on Histological Grade

Characteristic	High Grade	Low Grade
Estrogen receptors	Absent	Present
Comedo features	Present	Infrequent
Ploidy	Aneuploid	Diploid
Proliferative rate	High	Low
Her-2/neu	Overexpression	Normal copies
p53 mutation	Present	Absent
Calcification found on mammography	Coarse	Fine granular
Microinvasion	Present	Infrequent
Microvascular density	High	Low

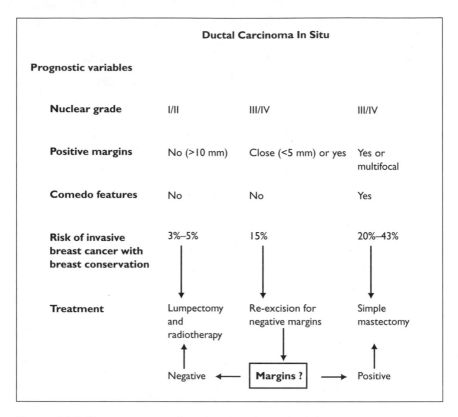

Figure 12-2 Treatment approach to ductal carcinoma in situ.

quency of relapse in patients with high-grade DCIS is 20% to 43% at 5 years.

The treatment approach is shown in Figure 12-2. Ductal carcinoma in situ is an almost 100% curable cancer (the true cures rate is 99% at 10 years), and the focus of therapy should be a curative outcome, even if it means a simple mastectomy is necessary. Breast reconstruction is always an option for women who require simple mastectomy.

Invasive Breast Cancer Treatment and Prognosis

The treatment of women with invasive breast cancer is based on the clinical and pathologic stage (see Table 12-1) and on the other important prognostic variables such as tumor size, patient age, menopausal status, estrogen and progesterone receptor status, and overexpression of the *Her-2/neu* gene. For women with breast cancers less than 5 cm in size (stages I and II), lumpectomy, axillary sampling, and breast irradiation (breast conservation) are equivalent to a modified radical mastectomy. The choice of either of these two treatment methods is influenced by the age of the patient, the size and location of the breast cancer (women with subareolar cancers are not candidates for breast conservation), the size of the breast, and the possible cosmetic outcome with breast conservation.

The lumpectomy specimen should include the entire breast cancer and a rim of at least 5 mm of normal breast tissue. There should not be any microscopic extension into a margin. If there is, a re-excision needs to be performed. Patients with multifocal breast cancer or with continued positive margins on re-excision are not candidates for breast conservation. The axillary sampling is, simply put, just that—a sampling. The sample should include at least 15 to 16 lymph nodes. The nodes sampled are the level 1 and 2 nodes. A complete axillary dissection can injure the axillary vein and lead to edema of the arm. Furthermore, more extensive axillary dissections do not provide more information than limited axillary sampling. From a treatment and prognosis standpoint, the axillary sampling informs the physician as to whether the nodes are uninvolved or involved and the number that harbor metastases (1–3, 4–9, >10). Breast cancer does not ascend the level 1 and 2 lymph nodes like rungs of a ladder. The level 1 nodes may be uninvolved, and there may be involvement of nodes at level 2. However, despite care and an axillary dissection of level 1 and 2 nodes, lymphedema develops in approximately 9% to 10% of women.

Recently, an axillary sampling procedure called *sentinel node biopsy* has undergone initial evaluation in women with stages I and II breast cancer in an attempt to avoid lymphedema and more extensive axillary sampling. In this procedure, technetium-99 sulfur colloid is injected subdermally into the skin a few millimeters away from the breast mass in a circular pattern. The surgeon then waits sometimes as long as 1 to 2 hours and with a hand-held gamma camera determines the amount of uptake in the axilla. The "sentinel nodes," usually one or two axillary lymph nodes that show the greatest uptake, are excised and sent for frozen section. If the nodes show no evidence of metastatic involvement, the axillary incision is closed and the surgeon proceeds with the lumpectomy. If metastases are found on frozen section, the axillary sampling is completed (a level 1 and 2 node dissection) to determine the number of nodes involved. The sentinel node biopsy procedure is still regarded by some surgeons as experimental, and there is controversy about the use of this procedure. In experienced hands, a sentinel node biopsy that shows no metastatic involvement carries a true-negative rate of 95% to 96% and a false-negative rate of 4%.

The treatment of women with stages I and II breast cancer is shown in Table 12-3. Women with stage I breast cancer overall have an excellent prog-

Table 12-3 Treatment of Stages I and II Breast Cancer

Stage	Local Therapy	Adjunctive Chemotherapy	Disease-Free Survival at 10 Years (%)
Stage I			
T<5 mm	BC or MRM	None	92–95
T 5–9 mm	BC or MRM	None	92–95
T >10 mm ER+	BC or MRM	Tamoxifen	87–89
T >10 mm ER–, <49	BC or MRM	CMF or MF	83–85
T >10 mm ER–, >49	BC or MRM	CMF or MF	83–85
Stage II			
Node negative, ER–	BC or MRM	Clinical trial or CMF or AC	72–80
Node negative, ER+ or PR+	BC or MRM	Clinical trial or tamoxifen +/– CMF	75–82
Node positive <10, ER–, <49 or >49 y	BC or MRM	Clinical trial or AC + paclitaxel	65–73 projected at 5 y
Node positive <10, ER+ or PR+, <49 y	BC or MRM	Clinical trial or AC + paclitaxel	65–73 projected at 5 y
Node positive <10, ER+ or PR+, >49 y	BC or MRM	Clinical trial or AC + paclitaxel followed by tamoxifen	65–73 projected at 5 y
Node positive >10, ER+ or ER–, any age	BC or MRM	Clinical trial or AC + paclitaxel +/– tamoxifen if ER+	40–52 at 5 y
Node positive >10 with *Her-2/neu* overexpression	BC or MRM	Clinical trial	35–40 at 5 y

T = tumor; ER = estrogen receptor; PR = progesterone receptor; BC = breast conservation, lumpectomy, axillary sampling, radiation therapy; MRM = modified radical mastectomy; CMF = cyclophosphamide, methotrexate, and 5-fluorouracil; MF = methotrexate with leucovorin rescue and 5-fluorouracil; AC = Adriamycin (doxorubicin) and cyclophosphamide.

nosis and often require no adjunctive chemotherapy. The prognosis and treatment approach to women with stage II breast cancer varies with their menopausal status (arbitrarily subdivided as premenopausal for women younger than 49 years of age and as postmenopausal for women older than 49 years of age), the presence of estrogen or progesterone receptors (ER/PR), and the number of involved lymph nodes. Women with stage II, node-negative breast cancer should receive adjunctive therapy as shown in Table 12-3. Women with stage II, node-negative breast cancer that is ER-positive should receive adjuvant tamoxifen alone or in combination with CMF (cytoxan, methotrexate, 5-fluorouracil) chemotherapy. Women with stage II, node-negative breast cancer that is ER-negative should receive adjuvant CMF chemotherapy. Women with stage II, node-positive breast cancer, regardless of whether the breast cancer is ER-positive or ER-negative and whether the patient is premenopausal or postmenopausal, should receive adjuvant chemotherapy with Adriamycin (doxorubicin) and cyclophosphamide (AC) every 3 weeks for 12 weeks followed by paclitaxel (Taxol) every 3 weeks for 12 weeks. A large randomized study has compared two dose schedules of AC with or without Taxol (1). The early results of this trial showed a statistically significant improvement in disease-free and overall survival at 18 months for the group receiving AC followed by Taxol. Women who have ER-positive breast cancer should receive tamoxifen in addition to AC followed by Taxol. Women with stage II, node-positive breast cancer with more than 10 lymph nodes involved have a particularly poor prognosis and should be encouraged to participate in clinical trials.

Case 12-1

A 78-year-old white woman was seen for a second opinion with regard to the treatment of a very recent diagnosis of breast cancer. She had found a lump in her right breast 4 weeks earlier and had seen her internist, who ordered a mammogram. Mammography showed a 2-cm mass in the right medial upper quadrant of the breast consistent with breast cancer. She was then referred to a surgeon. The surgeon performed a core biopsy, and the histopathologic findings indicated an invasive infiltrating ductal breast cancer. A lumpectomy and axillary sampling were planned but were subsequently canceled because a 2-cm mass was found in the right middle lobe on chest radiography. Computed tomography (CT) of the chest showed a 3-cm mass in the right middle lobe surrounded by lung with emphysematous changes. No hilar or mediastinal lymphadenopathy was present; no other pulmonary nodules were present. A CT-guided fine-needle aspiration (FNA) revealed adenocarcinoma, and the patient was referred to a medical oncologist who deemed that she had stage IV disease and advised chemotherapy. Her past medical history was significant for chronic bronchitis. She was a smoker in excess of 60 pack years.

The physical findings revealed a 2.5-cm right breast mass at the 2 o'clock position with a resolving ecchymosis. No clinically palpable adenopathy was present. The lung examination revealed inspiratory rhonchi with a slight prolongation of the expiratory phase. The remainder of the physical examination was unremarkable. Review of the CT scan of the chest showed the 3-cm right middle lobe mass without associated adenopathy or other pulmonary nodules. A bone scan was obtained that showed solely degenerative changes, and findings of CT of the brain were normal. Serum markers CEA and AC 27.29 were both within normal limits. Pathologic review of the FNA and the breast core biopsy showed adenocarcinomas that ap-

Continued.

Case 12-1—cont'd

peared slightly different. Immunohistochemistry on the breast core biopsy showed expression of ER and PR and no overexpression of *Her-2/neu*. Immunohisto-chemistries could not be done on the FNA of the lung mass owing to inadequate material. *The conclusion reached based on the work-up was that of two separate primaries—one in the lung and the other in the breast—based on the histologic appearance and the lack of metastatic involvement elsewhere.*

The patient had pulmonary function testing and subsequently a radical mastectomy and lobectomy, and at the same setting, a lumpectomy and right axillary sampling. She was found to have an unequivocal stage IB adenocarcinoma of the right lung (pathologic T2 N0 M0) and a stage II node-negative breast cancer. She began treatment with adjuvant tamoxifen, 10 mg orally twice daily, and after her recovery, radiation therapy was administered to the right breast.

Women with stage IIIA breast cancer (tumor >5 cm) can be treated in two ways. One way is to proceed with a modified radical mastectomy (MRM) and then make decisions as to adjunctive therapy based on the ER status and the number of nodes involved, as in the case of patients with stage II cancer. Postoperative radiotherapy should be delivered to the chest wall, because these patients are at high risk for local recurrence. The other approach to patients with stage IIIA cancer is to administer neoadjuvant chemotherapy AC alone (12 weeks) or AC followed by treatment with paclitaxel (24 weeks), bearing in mind that in more than 90% of patients the tumor regresses and that in 16% to 30% the tumor disappears completely without any trace pathologically. Neoadjuvant chemotherapy may allow breast conservation and spare patients with stage IIIA cancer having to undergo an MRM. The drawback to neoadjuvant chemotherapy is that the physician will never actually know the number of lymph nodes involved at the onset, because in most cases there will be a significant down-staging of the axillary lymph nodes. After neoadjuvant chemotherapy is completed and provided that the patient has had a good response to treatment (CR [complete response, or, complete clinical disappearance] or PR [>50% reduction in the surface area]), a lumpectomy with axillary sampling (a sentinel node biopsy is contraindicated) and breast irradiation complete the treatment. Additional chemotherapy may be needed in some women treated with this approach. The overall results in stage IIIA cancer are a disease-free survival at 5 years of 54% to 70%.

The toxicities of both adjuvant and neoadjuvant chemotherapy vary with the regimen. CMF and MF are not highly emetogenic regimens, and the acute hematologic toxicities with these regimens are relatively mild. Neutropenic fever is an infrequent occurrence. Some women report weight gain with CMF, presumably as a result of cyclophosphamide-induced gastric irritation that improves with meals. Doxorubicin-based regimens (AC, AC-Taxol) carry a greater risk of neutropenic fever and greater hematologic toxicities. In addition, such regimens carry the risk of treatment-induced leukemia (<1%). The treatment-induced leukemias from doxorubicin are usually myelomonocytic and have abnormalities of chromosome 11. Other potential toxicities include a 1% risk of deep venous thrombosis and treatment-induced amenorrhea. The acute toxicities from breast irradiation include erythema of the breast or chest wall that infrequently evolves to frank skin desquamation, edema of the breast (the typical symptom is chest heaviness), and, occasionally, cough. Long-term toxicities usually begin to manifest 6 to 9 months after the breast or chest wall irradiation is completed; these include arm edema (5% to 20%), rib fractures (5%), radiation-induced brachial plexopathy (1%), second malignancies other than breast cancer (<0.1%), and poor cosmetic outcomes (5%). Toxicities from tamoxifen include weight gain, hot flashes, deep venous thrombosis (2%), and endometrial cancer (0.4%).

Women who receive therapy for breast cancer are at a 3% risk of recurrence of breast cancer in the irradiated breast and a 14% risk of contralateral breast cancer. Provided that there is no evidence of metastases, the treatment of recurrent breast cancer in an irradiated breast is mastectomy. Breast reconstruction is difficult but not impossible in this setting. Patients who wish to have breast reconstruction should be referred to a plastic surgeon skilled in microvascular surgery.

The treatment approach to women with inflammatory breast cancer stage IIIB is similar to that used in women with stage IIIA disease—namely, initial chemotherapy with AC followed by Taxol, and subsequently mastectomy followed by radiation therapy, which is in turn followed by additional chemotherapy. Women who overexpress *Her-2/neu* are candidates for Herceptin, the murine monoclonal anti-*Her-2/neu* receptor antibody. Women with inflammatory breast cancer may be candidates for clinical trials exploring high-dose chemotherapy with autologous bone marrow transplantation (ABMT), which is under investigation at the present time. The median time to treatment failure for these women is 24 to 36 months; the disease-free survival at 5 years is 30% to 45%, with an overall 5-year survival of 55%.

The treatment of women with stage IV breast cancer is clearly palliative. Although some do extraordinarily well, ostensibly with no clinical evidence of disease, we do not consider that they have been "cured" of breast cancer. Relapse is likely even 5 and 10 years after the attainment of a complete response. Three questions need to be answered to determine the course of palliation of stage IV breast cancer:

1. Is the breast cancer hormonally responsive (does it express ER and/or PR)?
2. Where are the dominant metastatic sites (e.g., skin/chest wall/nodal, lung, liver, bone, multiple visceral)?
3. Does the breast cancer overexpress/amplify the *Her-2/neu* gene product/gene?

In premenopausal or postmenopausal women with ER-positive and PR-positive, ER-negative and PR-positive, or ER/PR unknown breast cancer metastatic to bone, chest wall, or lung but without multiple liver or lymphangitic metastasis, an initial trial of hormone therapy (6 weeks) is appropriate. In this non–life-threatening setting, the physician has time to evaluate the response to hormone therapy. If hormone therapy is effective as judged by either a greater than 50% reduction in the surface area (greatest tumor diameter and its perpendicular) of all measurable lesions or a decline in tumor markers (see Chapter 2, p 42) in patients with bone-only disease, this then opens "the sequential hormonal treatment pathway" as shown in Figure 12-3. Even if their cancer is ER-positive and PR-positive, patients with either hepatic metastases or lymphangitic pulmonary metastases have life-threatening stage IV breast cancer, and the physician therefore does not have the luxury of time to determine the responsiveness or lack of responsiveness to hormonal therapy. In this situation, chemotherapy is indicated.

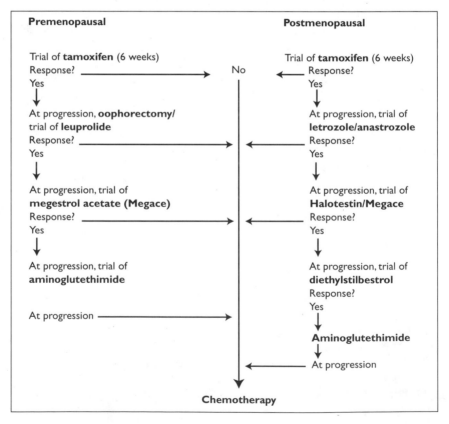

Figure 12-3 Sequential hormonal treatment pathway for stage IV breast cancer.

The probability of response to tamoxifen is 30% to 40% for women who are either ER-positive or PR-positive, but 70% for women who are both ER-positive and PR-positive. The median duration of tamoxifen-induced response (complete or partial) is 9 to 12 months. Subsequent hormonal therapy usually leads to the probability of response at a rate of 25% to 35%, and a median duration of response of 5 to 6 months.

The toxicities of hormonal therapy include hot flashes, deep vein thrombosis, uterine cancer (tamoxifen), weight gain, edema, uterine bleeding, hypertension (megestrol acetate [Megace]), hot flashes and hair loss (letrozole, anastrozole), masculinization and liver function abnormalities (Halotestin), skin rashes, agranulocytosis, and adrenal insufficiency (aminoglutethimide). The following case (Case 12-2) illustrates the potential benefits of hormone therapy in the treatment of women with stage IV breast cancer.

Case 12-2

A 60-year-old woman presented to her internist with a complaint of a lump on her forehead. She had been in her usual state of health until 3 month earlier when she first noted the lump, which over the next 3 months increased in size and became painful. She denied any trauma, other lumps or masses, any myalgias, arthralgias, or bone pain. Her past medical history was significant for hypertension and type II diabetes mellitus that she controlled with diet alone. Her medication included hydrochlorothiazide and K-Lyte.

The relevant physical findings revealed a 3 × 3 cm firm mass palpable on her forehead and a large ulcerated 7 × 7 cm mass in the left breast. A large 2 × 3 cm lymph nodal mass was palpable in the left axilla. A core biopsy of the left breast mass was consistent with breast cancer. An FNA of the forehead mass revealed an adenocarcinoma consistent with breast cancer. A bone scan showed widespread bone metastases to the ribs, thoracic spine, skull, and pelvis. The ER and PR content of the breast mass revealed high levels of both ER and PR. The patient began treatment with tamoxifen and underwent a palliative left MRM to avoid complications of cellulitis and/or bleeding.

Her response to tamoxifen as judged by the forehead mass was dramatic, with complete regression of the mass in the forehead. She has been taking tamoxifen for the past 10 years, and last year began treatment with letrozole because of progressive bone disease. She continues to work full-time at age 71 years, and she is in her eleventh year with stage IV breast cancer.

Discussion
This woman's response to tamoxifen was dramatic and her duration of response exceeds the median many times over. Clearly, her breast cancer is biologically indolent; however, the magnitude and degree of palliation by hormone therapy are impressive.

Women with stage IV breast cancer who are ER/PR–negative, who have liver metastases or lymphangitic pulmonary metastases, or who do not respond to hormone therapy are candidates for combination chemotherapy. If a clinical trial is available, they should be encouraged to participate. AC and CMF are both effective regimens. Other chemotherapy regimens include cyclophosphamide, mitoxantrone, and 5-fluorouracil (CNF) and Navelbine (vinorelbine), 5-fluorouracil, and leucovorin (NFL).

The probability of response to these regimens varies from 50% to 70%, with a median response duration of 9 to 15 months. The median survival is more a function of the dominant metastatic sites than is the regimen used (Table 12-4). The toxicities of such regimens primarily include myelosuppression, mucositis, diarrhea, hair loss, fatigue, and cardiomyopathy (AC, CNF). In women who respond to treatment and then develop disease progression after the use of an initial regimen (CMF, AC, CNF, and NFL) or who do not respond to initial treatment, the use of a taxane (paclitaxel [Taxol] or docetaxel [Taxotere]) is indicated. Although comparative trials between paclitaxel and docetaxel have not been conducted, either drug has a 45% probability of inducing an objective response in this setting. The response duration to the taxanes is 7 to 9 months. Toxicities include hypersensitive reactions to paclitaxel, which are treated prophylactically with steroids (dexamethasone [Decadron]), myalgias, peripheral neuropathy, myelosuppression (docetaxel), and peripheral edema of uncertain cause, which is prevented by the prophylactic use of steroids (dexamethasone). Patients who ultimately progress after treatment with taxanes are candidates for either phase II clinical trials or capecitabine (Xeloda), a fluorouracil analogue that is administered orally if their performance status is good. For women with poor performance status, palliative treatment is most appropriate. The probability of response to capecitabine is 20%, with a median response duration of 6 months. Capecitabine must be dosed cautiously because of its toxicities, which include

Table 12-4 Median Survival in Stage IV Breast Cancer as a Function of the Dominant Metastatic Sites

Dominant Metastatic Sites	Median Survival (mo)
Skin, chest wall, nodal	>40
Pleural effusion only	36
Bone, single site	40–48
Bone, multiple sites	24
Pulmonary, nonlymphangitic	18
Liver	12
Brain only	18–24
Disseminated visceral	9–12

myelosuppression, ataxia, diarrhea, mucositis, and hand-and-foot syndrome. The use of high-dose chemotherapy with ABMT in stage IV breast cancer continues to be investigational. One small South African randomized trial showed a potential benefit (2). In stark contrast a large American trial showed absolutely no benefit to ABMT in the stage IV setting (3). It is likely that ABMT will have a very limited or no role at all in the palliation of women with stage IV breast cancer. Other trials that have concluded accrual are pending at this time.

An important adjunctive treatment in women who have breast cancer with predominantly bone involvement is the use of pamidronate (Aredia), which has been shown in a randomized clinical trial to decrease the probability of fracture by 50% in women with stage IV breast cancer and bone metastases (4, 5).

Women with stage IV breast cancer and *Her-2/neu* overexpression are candidates for chemotherapy and the concurrent use of Herceptin (a humanized murine, anti-*Her-2/neu* receptor monoclonal antibody). Although the exact pathophysiology at a molecular level has not been fully elucidated, the in vitro data show that breast cancer cell lines that overamplify the *Her-2/neu* gene are resistant to the killing effects of chemotherapeutic drugs, with the possible exception of the taxanes. The clinical data certainly suggest that women with stage IV breast cancer and *Her-2/neu* overexpression have an extremely aggressive form of this disease.

A randomized trial in women with stage IV breast cancer compared AC with and without Herceptin, and paclitaxel with and without Herceptin (6). The study showed a benefit to the use of Herceptin, with the greatest impact seen in the paclitaxel trial. However, Herceptin must be used with caution, because when used alone the antibody can cause cardiomyopathy (9% incidence). When Herceptin was used with AC, the incidence increased to 13%, which is much higher than the base incidence of 2% to 3% seen with the use of AC alone. The ejection fraction needs to be closely monitored in women receiving Herceptin in combination with either AC or Taxol. It is recommended that in women receiving AC and Herceptin, the total dose of doxorubicin should not exceed 350 mg/m^2.

Having entered the era of molecular medicine, we should have little doubt that we will be using a wide array of treatments aimed at molecular products or end points in women with breast cancer. The future looks increasingly bright.

REFERENCES

1. **Henderson IC, Berry D, Demetri G, et al.** Improved disease-free (DFS) and overall survival (OS) from the addition of sequential paclitaxel (T) but not from the escalation of doxorubicin (A) dose level in the adjuvant chemotherapy of patients with node pos-

itive breast cancer. Proceedings of American Society of Clinical Oncology. 1998;17: 101a (abstract 390).

2. **Bezwoda WR, Seymour L, Dansey RD.** High-dose chemotherapy and hematopoietic rescue as primary treatment for metastatic breast cancer: a randomized trial. J Clin Oncol. 1995;13:2483–9.

3. **Stadtmauer EA, O'Neill A, Golstein LW, et al.** Phase III randomized trial of high-dose chemotherapy and stem cell support shows no difference in overall survival or severe toxicity compared to maintenance chemotherapy with cyclophosphamide, methotrexate, and 5-fluorouracil (CMF) for women with metastatic breast cancer who are responding to conventional induction therapy. The Philadlephia Intergroup Study. Proceedings of the American Society of Clinical Oncology. 1999;18:1a (abstract 1).

4. **Hortobagyi GN, Theriault RL, Porter L, et al.** Efficacy of pamidronate in reducing skeletal complications in patients with breast cancer and lytic bone metastases. Protocol 19 Aredia Breast Cancer Study Group. N Engl J Med. 1996;335:1785–91.

5. **Theriault RL, Lipton A, Hortobagyi GN, et al.** Pamidronate reduces skeletal morbidity in women with advanced breast cancer and lytic bone lesions: a randomized, placebo-controlled trial. Protocol 18 Aredia Breast Cancer Study Group. J Clin Oncol. 1999;17:846–54.

6. **Slamon D, Leyland-Jones B, Shank S, et al.** Addition of Herceptin (humanized anti-*Her2* antibody) to first-line chemotherapy for *Her2* overexpressing metastatic breast cancer (*Her2*+/MBC) markedly increases anticancer activity: a randomized, multinational, controlled phase III trial. Proceedings of the American Society of Clinical Oncology. 1998;17:98a (abstract 377).

Chapter 13

Melanoma, Sarcoma, Central Nervous System Malignancies, and Unknown Primary Malignancies

Melanoma

Melanoma is an increasingly common malignancy in the United States, probably as a result of a thinning ozone layer that in the past has filtered out ultraviolet radiation. The incidence of melanoma has increased particularly in the Southwest, where the incidence is now 20 cases per 100,000 persons. In contrast, the incidence in the northern region of the United States is unchanged at 12 cases per 100,000 persons. Melanoma has a bimodal incidence, affecting young persons 20 to 30 years old, and reaching another peak at 55 to 60 years of age. In fact, melanoma is the most common cancer in women 25 to 29 years old. Risk factors for melanoma are ultraviolet light exposure, fair skin, and a family history (dysplastic nevus syndrome; see Table 1-6, p 17).

Signs and Symptoms

Patients with melanoma may be asymptomatic or they may report that a "mole has changed." The physical examination should be performed with a completely disrobed patient in a well-lit room, and nevi should be thoroughly evaluated for changes suggestive of early melanoma (asymmetry, border irregularity, color, and diameter) (Table 13-1). Examples of early melanomas are shown in Figure 13-1. Patients who are considered at risk for melanoma, patients who have already been diagnosed with melanoma, and patients and

Table 13-1 Characteristics of Benign Mole versus Melanoma

Mole	Color	Borders	Symmetry	Diameter
Benign mole	Uniform Tan	Regular	Symmetrical	< 6 mm
Melanoma	Variegated	Irregular	Asymmetrical	> 6 mm

family members identified with dysplastic nevus syndrome should be referred to multispecialty melanoma screening clinics where nevi are mapped and photographed and where the person at risk is closely followed.

If a suspicious lesion is identified, it should be completely excised. Shave biopsies should be avoided. The staging of melanoma takes into account the thickness of the primary lesion as determined by Breslow thickness, the presence or absence of lymphadenopathy, and the presence or absence of metastases (Table 13-2). The thickness of the melanoma is categorized as follows: less than 0.75 mm, 0.76 to 1.50 mm, 1.51 to 4.0 mm, and greater than 4.0 mm.

Treatment

The treatment of melanoma is surgical excision. If the melanoma is less than 1 mm in thickness, a 1-cm margin should be obtained. If the melanoma is 1 to 4 mm thick, the excisional margin should be 2 cm. If the melanoma is greater than 4 mm thick, the margin around the melanoma should be at least 2 cm. If the margins of resection are involved, a re-excision is mandatory.

The issue of lymphadenectomy is controversial. The probability of nodal metastases is a function of the thickness of the melanoma (Table 13-3). Therefore, the current recommendation is that if the melanoma is less than 1 mm thick, a wide excision without lymphadenectomy is all that is required. If the melanoma is 1 to 4 mm thick and no palpable lymphadenopathy is present, a wide excision with a 2-cm margin is recommended and a lymphadenectomy is not required. Rather, the patient should be watched and, if lymphadenopathy develops, the lymph nodes can be excised at that time. Studies examining prophylactic lymphadenectomy compared with delayed lymphadenectomy have not shown a survival benefit to prophylactic lymphadenectomy. If the melanoma is greater than 4 mm thick, a sentinel node biopsy is recommended, and if positive for metastatic involvement, a lymphadenectomy should be performed. The procedure of sentinel node biopsy is identical to that used in women with breast cancer (see Chapter 12, p 199). Patients with melanoma and palpable lymph nodes (stage III) are best treated with wide excision and lymphadenectomy. Patients with stage II (T4, >4 mm thick) and stage III melanoma are candidates for adjuvant chemotherapy with recombi-

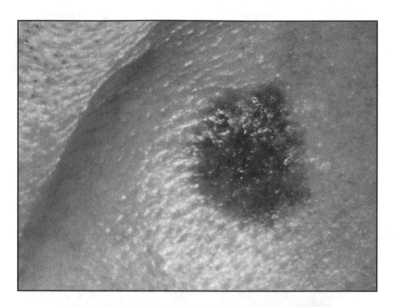

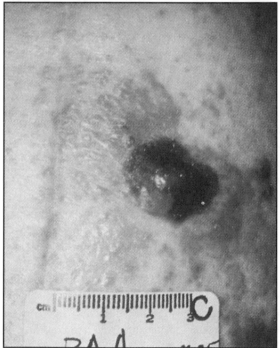

Figure 13-1 Two early melanomas. Note the differences in shading and irregular borders.

Table 13-2 Staging of Melanoma

Tumor		Nodes		Metastases	
T1	<0.75 mm	N0	No nodal involvement	M0	No metastases
T2	0.76–1.50 mm	N1	Regional nodal metastases	M1	Presence of distant metastases
T3	1.51–4.0 mm				
T4	>4.0 mm				

Stage	
I	T1, N0, M0 or T2, N0, M0
II	T3, N0, M0 or T4, N0, M0
III	Any T, N1, M0
IV	Any T, any N, M1

Table 13-3 Probability of Nodal Metastases Based on the Thickness of Melanoma

Tumor	Breslow Thickness	Probability of Nodal Involvement
T1	<0.75 mm	<5%
T2	0.76–1.50 mm	5%–10%
T3	1.51–4.0 mm	20%–25%
T4	>4 mm	35%

nant α-interferon. A randomized trial in patients with stage II and stage III melanoma showed a survival benefit for patients receiving interferon (1). The interferon treatment is rigorous, because the dose and schedule are high (20 million U 5 days per week for 4 weeks, then 10 million U subcutaneously three times per week for 48 weeks). Patients with stage IV melanoma may participate in a clinical trial or can be palliated with chemoimmunotherapy or immunotherapy alone. Although there is a dearth of randomized trials in stage IV melanoma, the results of chemoimmunotherapy appear promising. Table 13-4 summarizes the treatment and outcome on a stage-by-stage basis.

Sarcoma

Osteogenic and soft tissue sarcomas are extremely rare cancers. Together they may account for approximately 11,000 cancers per year. The median age of onset for soft tissue sarcoma is 50 to 60 years. In contrast, osteogenic sarcoma is a disease of childhood and adolescents. The risk factor for soft tissue sarcoma is previous radiotherapy, previous use of alkylating agents, and expo-

Table 13-4 Treatment of Melanoma

Stage	Treatment	5-year Relapse-Free Survival (%)
I (T1)	Wide excision	90
I (T2)	Wide excision, 2 cm margin	90
II (T3)	Wide excision, 2 cm margin	70
II (T4)	Wide excision, with at least 2 cm margin; sentinel node biopsy; if biopsy for metastatic involvement, lymphadenectomy, adjuvant interferon	60–65
III (N1)	Wide excision, with at least 2 cm margin; lymphadenectomy and adjuvant interferon	45–50
IV	Clinical trial or palliative chemoimmunotherapy or immunotherapy	5–10

sure to phenoxyacetic acid or vinyl chloride. The risk factor for osteogenic sarcoma is hereditary retinoblastoma; other risk factors are unknown.

Signs and Symptoms

The signs and symptoms of soft tissue sarcoma vary with the location in the extremity. Patients usually note a painless mass; retroperitoneal sarcomas produce few symptoms until they are quite large. Osteogenic sarcoma usually causes extremity pain and swelling. Studies that should be done include radiography, and if the results raise suspicion, magnetic resonance imaging (MRI). The physical findings are either a mass in the extremity or an abdominal mass. The presence of a mass more than 5 cm and persistent for longer than 4 to 6 weeks mandates a biopsy.

In the case of soft tissue sarcoma, the biopsy should be excision. In the case of osteogenic sarcoma, an incisional biopsy or needle biopsy is all that is required.

A patient with any type of sarcoma should be evaluated by a multidisciplinary group involving medical oncologists, radiation oncologists, orthopedic surgeons, surgical oncologists, and pathologists.

Treatment

The treatment of osteogenic sarcoma is much different than that of soft tissue sarcomas. Patients with osteogenic sarcoma should be referred to a center that has a multidisciplinary group on site (orthopedic surgeons with a specialty in sarcoma, medical oncologists, pathologists, prosthetic specialists, radiation oncologists) able to handle this highly complex disease. Patients with osteogenic sarcoma are best treated with neoadjuvant chemotherapy, fol-

Table 13-5 Staging of Soft Tissue Sarcoma

Tumor Grade (G)		Tumor Size		Nodes		Metastases	
1	Well differentiated	T1	<5cm	N0	None	M0	Present
2	Moderately differentiated	T2	>5cm	N1	Nodal	M1	Absent
3	Poorly differentiated				metastases		
4	Undifferentiated						

Stage	
IA	G1, T1, N0, M0
IB	G1, T2, N0, M0
IIA	G2, T1, N0, M0
IIB	G2, T2, N0, M0
IIIA	G3 or G4, T1, N0, M0
IIIB	G3 or G4, T2, N0, M0
IVA	Any G, any T, N1, M0
IVB	Any G, any T, any N, M1

lowed by limb-sparing surgery, followed by additional chemotherapy. The resultant 5- and 10-year disease-free survival in patients with osteogenic sarcoma is 74% to 78%.

Patients with soft tissue sarcomas are treated with wide surgical excision. If an extremity requires amputation, it is preferable to attempt wide excision followed by radiation therapy in an attempt to spare the limb. Adjuvant chemotherapy has no established role. The staging system of soft tissue sarcomas is shown in Table 13-5.

The results of surgical therapy in patients with soft tissue sarcoma are highly dependent on stage and can vary from 90% 5-year disease-free survival rates for patients with stage IA liposarcoma to 35% for patients with stage IIIA malignant fibrous histiocytomas. Patients with large retroperitoneal sarcomas that are not amenable to surgery can be palliated with radiotherapy.

Patients with sarcomas metastatic to lung may be candidates for surgical resection or can be palliated with ifosfamide/doxorubicin–based chemotherapy regimens.

Central Nervous System Malignancies

Most primary central nervous system (CNS) malignancies are neuroectodermal tumors that arise from the glial cells (gliomas) and are subcategorized as astrocytoma, anaplastic astrocytoma, oligodendrogliomas, glioblastoma multiforme (characterized by necrosis and endothelial proliferation), and primitive neuroectodermal tumors (PNET). Primary CNS lymphomas account for fewer than 5%

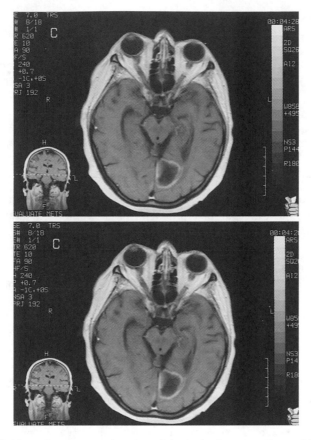

Figure 13-2 Magnetic resonance imaging of the brain demonstrating multiple ring enhancing masses. The largest mass is in the left optical lobe and measures 3 cm in diameter. Perifocal edema is present. There is no midline shift. The masses represent metastatic adenocarcinoma of the lung.

of all CNS tumors. The incidence of primary CNS tumors in the United States is 9.5 per 100,000 persons. Risk factors for malignant gliomas include tuberous sclerosis, neurofibromatosis, Li-Fraumeni syndrome, and Turcot syndrome. The signs and symptoms of primary CNS tumors are nonspecific and include nausea and vomiting (caused by increased intracranial pressure), headache, seizures, a strokelike presentation, and hemiparesis. The MRI and/or infused computed tomography (CT) are almost diagnostic of a CNS malignancy, which typically demonstrates an intracranial mass with edema (Fig. 13-2). After a solitary mass has been identified, the physician must determine whether this mass represents a primary CNS tumor as opposed to a solitary CNS metastasis. To facilitate this differential, a thorough physical examination is repeated and chest radiography, multi-channel chemistries, a complete blood count, and a urinalysis are done. In the meantime, the patient begins treatment with dexamethasone, loading dose of 8 mg IVP, followed by 4 mg orally every 6 hours with the dose titrated to control symptoms. The patient should also begin treatment with prophylactic phenytoin (Dilantin) 300 to 400 mg/d with therapeutic monitoring of the Dilantin levels. A neurosurgeon is consulted for a biopsy, possibly stereotactic depending on the location of the tumor. The subsequent treatment decisions are based on the histology of the tumor.

For low-grade gliomas, astrocytoma grades I and II, all that is required is neurosurgical resection alone. Low-grade gliomas have a tendency to recur and transform into higher-grade gliomas. In patients with higher-grade gliomas, astrocytoma (grades III/IV), anaplastic astrocytoma, and glioblastoma multiforme, the treatment approach is limited resection and whole brain radiation therapy to at least 60 Gy followed by chemotherapy with procarbazine, CCNU, and vincristine (PCV). The median survival for patients with anaplastic astrocytoma treated in this manner is 18 months, with a 2-year survival of 30% to 40%. The median survival for patients with glioblastoma multiforme is 10 to 12 months with a 2-year survival of 20%.

Primitive neuroectodermal tumors are high-grade, aggressive tumors that usually occur in childhood. When they occur in the cerebellum, they are identified as medulloblastoma; elsewhere in the CNS, the term PNET is used. The treatment of PNET and medulloblastoma is surgical resection, craniospinal radiotherapy to 36 Gy, followed by chemotherapy (cyclophosphamide, vincristine, CCNU, and cisplatin). The 5-year survival is 60%.

Primary CNS lymphoma is increasing in incidence both in the general population as well as in the population at risk—namely, persons infected with human immunodeficiency virus. The treatment is chemotherapy with a high-dose methotrexate-containing regimen and whole brain radiotherapy.

The management of brain metastases is predicated on whether the lesion is a solitary metastasis or multiple and whether metastases exist elsewhere. If there are multiple brain metastases or metastases to other sites, the treatment is palliative and consists of dexamethasone, Dilantin, and whole brain irradiation to 45 to 50 Gy. If a solitary CNS metastasis exists without disease elsewhere and depending on the location of the metastasis, surgical resection may be warranted. A randomized trial has proven the superiority of neurosurgical resection over whole brain irradiation in this setting (2).

Patients with primary or metastatic CNS tumors that progress or re-grow after whole brain irradiation can be palliated with the use of radiosurgery. Radiosurgery is a technique of delivering a high dose of radiation, usually 10 to 20 Gy, one time to a confined and small volume. Radiosurgery can be delivered by either the gamma-knife (a misnomer because it is not actually a knife) or a linear accelerator. In this procedure, CT of the brain assists in the creation of a three-dimensional treatment plan. The patient is placed in a cradling device to keep the head still, and over the course of a few hours the radiation dose is delivered to the targeted area. Trials are underway to determine the role of radiosurgery as an initial treatment for CNS tumors.

Unknown Primary Malignancies

The definition of cancers of undetermined primary origin (CUP) and the diagnostic approach are reviewed in Chapter 2. Table 13-6 summarizes the cancers one needs to consider based on the presenting symptoms and physical findings. Cases occur in which after a careful history, physical examination, and prudent diagnostic studies the primary site cannot be found. Decisions regarding treatment approaches need to be made for these patients. Because there is no randomized study in CUP that compares best supportive care with a chemotherapy program and demonstrates a survival or quality of life advantage to chemotherapy, the approach that I use is a common sense one. If a patient is not particularly symptomatic or has a few symptoms that are easily controlled (i.e., pleurodesis of

Table 13-6 What to Consider in the Diagnostic Work-up of Selected Patients with Cancer of Unknown Primary Origin

Clinical Situation	Histology	Need to Rule Out	Next Steps
Young men or women with mediastinal or masses	Undifferentiated cancer	Extragonadal germ cell cancer	Serum AFP, β-HCG, stains for AFP and cytokeratin
Young men or women with pelvic masses	Undifferentiated cancer	Neuroblastoma	Urine HVA and VMA, cytogenetics
Women with cancer in axillary lymph nodes	Adenocarcinoma	Breast cancer	ER/PR, CA 27.29
Women with ascites	Adenocarcinoma	Ovarian cancer	ER/PR, CA-125
Men with bone or lung metastasis	Adenocarcinoma	Prostate cancer	Serum PSA, stain for PSA
Men or women with lung nodules, hilar or mediastinal masses	Adenocarcinoma	Lung cancer	Stain for cytokeratin
Men or women with single or multiple liver masses	Adenocarcinoma	Hepatoma	Serum AFP, CEA
Men or (rarely) women with enlarged cervical lymph nodes	Squamous cell cancer	Head and neck cancer	Stain for cytokeratin

AFP = α-fetoprotein; HCG = human chorionic gonadotropin; HVA = homovanillic acid; VMA = vanillylmandelic acid; ER = estrogen receptor; PR = progesterone receptor; PSA = prostate-specific antigen; CEA = carcinoembryonic antigen.

a malignant effusion, pain controlled by NSAIDs and/or narcotics), I simply follow the patient and wait for more severe symptoms to develop. In a patient who is symptomatic and has a good performance status, chemotherapy with carboplatin, etoposide, and paclitaxel (Taxol) is a treatment option. Patients with a poor performance status are best served by hospice care.

REFERENCES

1. **Kirkwood JM, Strawderman MH, Ernstoff MS, et al.** Interferon alpha-2b adjuvant therapy of high-risk resected cutaneous melanoma. The Eastern Cooperative Oncology Group Trial EST 1684. J Clin Oncol. 1996;14:7–17.
2. **Patchell RA, Tibbs PA, Walsh JW, et al.** A randomized trial of surgery in the treatment of single metastases to the brain. N Engl J Med. 1990;322:494–500.

Bibliography

Abeloff MD, Armitage JO, Litcher AS, Neiderhuber JE, eds. Clinical Oncology. New York: Churchill Livingston; 1995.

Bennett JM, Catovsky DM, et al. The French American British (FAB) Cooperative Group Proposals for the Chronic (Mature) B and T Lymphoid Leukemia. J Clin Pathol. 1989:567-84.

Bitran JD. Primary lung cancer. In: Rakel RE, ed. Conn's Current Therapy. Philadelphia: WB Saunders; 1998:189-95.

Bitran JD, Ultmann JE. The non-Hodgkin's lymphomas: presenting features. In: Magrath I, ed. The Non-Hodgkin's Lymphoma. 2nd ed. London: Edward Arnold; 1997:523-32.

Briasoulis E, Pavlidis N. Cancer of unknown primary origin. Oncologist. 1997;2:142-52.

Bruckman JE, Blommer WD. Management of spinal cord compression. Semin Oncol. 1978;5:135-40.

DeVita DT, Hellman S, Rosenberg SA, eds. Cancer: Principles and Practice of Oncology. 4th ed. Philadelphia: JB Lippincott; 1993.

Hesketh PJ, Kris MG, Grunberg SM, et al. Proposal for classifying the acute emetogenicity of cancer chemotherapy. J Clin Oncol. 1997;15:103-9.

Holland JF, Frei III E, Bast Jr RC, et al. Cancer Medicine. 4th ed. Baltimore: Williams & Wilkins; 1997.

Oesterling JE. Prostate-specific antigen: improving its ability to diagnose early prostate cancer. JAMA. 1992;267:2236-8.

Ohori M, Scardino PT. Early detection of prostate cancer: the nature of cancers detected with current diagnostic tests. Semin Oncol. 1994;21:522-6.

Pazdur R, Cola LR, Hoskins WJ, Wagman LD. Cancer Management: A Multidisciplinary Approach. 3rd ed. Melville, NY: Publisher Research & Representation; 1999.

Solomon D. Fine needle aspiration of the thyroid: an update. Thyroid Today. 1993;16:1-9.

Index

About the Author

D r. Jacob D. Bitran is a graduate of the University of Illinois College of Medicine. He completed his fellowship training at the University of Chicago. He was a faculty member of the University of Chicago from 1977 to 1991. Since 1991, he has been the Director of the Division of Hematology/Oncology at Lutheran General Hospital and Cancer Care Center, Park Ridge, Illinois.